Validation for Medical Device and Diagnostic Manufacturers

Carol DeSain

Charmaine Vercimak Sutton

Interpharm Press, Inc.
Buffalo Grove, IL

NEW BOOK CONCEPTS

Interpharm Press specializes in publishing books related to applied technology and regulatory affairs impacting the biotechnology, chemical, cosmetic, device, diagnostic or drug manufacturing industries. If you have a manuscript in progress, or are planning to write a book that will be applicable to development, medical, regulatory, manufacturing, quality or engineering professionals, please contact our editorial director.

SOCIAL RESPONSIBILITY PROGRAMS

Interpharm Resources Replenishment Program

Interpharm Press is significantly concerned with the worldwide loss of trees, and the impact of such loss on the environment and the availability of new drug sources. Losses to tropical rain forests are particularly remarkable in that only 3% of all possible endangered plant species have been evaluated for their active drug potential.

Interpharm Press commits to replant trees sufficient to replace those destroyed in meeting the paper needs for Interpharm's publications and advertising. Interpharm is actively supporting reforestation programs in Bangladesh, Israel, Kenya and the United States.

Pharmakos-2000

To foster the teaching of pharmaceutical technology, Interpharm Press has initiated its Pharmakos-2000 program. Under this program, one copy of this book is being sent, at no charge, to every College and School of Pharmacy worldwide. The program covers all 504 establishments listed by the Commonwealth Pharmaceutical Association (CPA) and the Federation Internationale Pharmaceutique (FIP).

It is hoped that this book will be a suitable reference resource to faculty and students advancing the theory and practice of pharmaceutical technology.

10 9 8 7 6 5 4 3 2

ISBN: 0-935184-64-3

Copyright © 1994 by Interpharm Press, Inc. All rights reserved.

Interpharm Press, Inc.
1358 Busch Parkway
Buffalo Grove, IL 60089, USA

Phone: + 1 + 708 + 459-8480
Fax: + 1 + 708 + 459-6644

Contents

8. Validation of Device Manufacturing in a One-Product Facility   71

Appendices

This book is dedicated to
the individuals who are responsible,
those who do the work, and
those who make the decisions.

Introduction

Validation is a fundamental building block that supports corporate commitments to quality assurance. Validation must be carefully planned to ensure that regulatory requirements are met and that corporate philosophies are maintained in a reasonable and cost-effective manner. Poorly planned and poorly understood commitments to validation can result in an excessive use of time and resources. Validation is **not** a product of the corporation; it is a tool of quality assurance.

Validation in medical device manufacturing is appropriate and often required in order to move a product from development to commercial production in the product life cycle. Validation confirms that product of predetermined quality and performance characteristics can be built reliably and reproducibly within established operating limits of the manufacturing process at the commercial manufacturing site.

The rigor and the complexity of the corporate commitment to validation is directly affected by the type of product and its use. Factors affecting when validation is appropriate include the following:

- The complexity or uniqueness of the product—its technology, its delivery system, or its packaging

- The critical nature of product usage (e.g., Class III Products vs. Class I Products; implantable vs. invasive vs. in vitro)

- The patient group affected (e.g., children, pregnant women, or AIDS patients vs. healthy adults)

- The setting in which the product is used (e.g., hospitals vs. home use)

The rigor and complexity of the corporate commitment to validation, similarly, is affected by the complexity and uniqueness of the manufacturing process and the manufacturing facility. For example,

- Is a single product manufactured in a dedicated manufacturing facility?

- Is a single product manufactured on a dedicated line in a facility with multiple products?

- Is the product manufactured on a campaign basis on a manufacturing line used for many products?

- Is the manufacturing process contracted out to one contractor?

- Is the manufacturing event contracted out to multiple contractors?

- Is the manufacturing technology unique?

- Is processing primarily manual?

- Is processing automated with custom-built equipment or software?

Where does one start? What are the basic requirements for validation? What is the difference between validation and qualification? How does one decide when validation is required? How much testing is enough? In this text we will apply the fundamentals of validation to product-specific manufacturing processes and to device manufacturing facilities that support multiple products. We will discuss how to plan a validation and how to make decisions about testing and also provide examples common among device manufacturers.

Chapter 1

<hr>

Quality Systems

The application of the principles of quality control, quality assurance, and validation in the medical product manufacturing industry has changed dramatically in the last 20 to 25 years. Consumer expectations and international competition have increased the pressures to produce goods of the highest quality at a reasonable cost. This expectation for the highest quality product at the most reasonable price must be balanced against another consumer edict: Medical products must be safe and effective at any cost.

Testing final product for compliance to predetermined specifications is no longer enough to assure quality. One must determine and control the quality of the raw materials for the manufacturing event and the quality of the manufacturing process. In the complex environment of the modern manufacturing facility with new technology products, assuring quality is a difficult task. Validation should be designed to maximize the assurance of quality and minimize testing.

For example, the raw materials for a manufacturing process include more than components and chemicals. Manufacturing equipment, test equipment, utility systems (water, air, steam, electric power), technicians, and the processing environment are also integral to the manufacturing process. To assure the quality of manufacturing processes, the quality of all components, equipment, technicians, and so on must be assured. The accepted practice for assuring the quality of the manufacturing process has been codified for medical product manufacturers in Title 21 of the *U.S. Code of Federal Regulations* as Good Manufacturing Practices (GMPs) since the 1970s. (Consult 21 CFR 210, 211, 600, 606, 820.)

The GMPs, however, are general expectations that each corporation must interpret in the context of its own product lines and its manufacturing facility. A manufacturer's interpretation of these expectations must be documented in corporate QA commitments, in procedures that describe how the commitments will be fulfilled, and in data collected to assure that the procedures have been implemented and the commitments fulfilled. These documents and this data must be accurate, authentic, complete, and available. The FDA will not give a manufacturer permission to distribute medical products in the U.S. market unless there is evidence that the product meets the manufacturer's standards for safety, performance, and reliability AND there is evidence of GMP compliance in the manufacturing facility.

The international community has additional quality assurance expectations for medical products manufacturers. The European Union will soon close its market to anyone who does not comply with harmonized standards and the quality systems of ISO 9000 as described in the *Essential Requirements of the Medical Device Directives.*

Manufacturers must interpret domestic and international expectations for quality assurance and develop corporate requirements that assure quality in the context of their product lines, their manufacturing facilities, and their markets. The quality assurance professional is responsible for ensuring that these expectations and requirements are fulfilled within the corporation.

So, how is this accomplished? What do you do first? And how do you know if you have missed something? The answer is to design a system that honors the basic principles of quality assurance and then ensure that those principles are honored at all levels in the system or organization.

Basic Principles of Quality Assurance

The four basic principles of quality assurance are as follows:

1. **Establish and confirm quality characteristics.** Know or determine what attributes or characteristics of an item, a process, or a product are important to its use, performance, or reliability. Establish methods to test for these attributes and determine a range of acceptable limits. Confirm that these specifications can be met routinely.

Validation, as presented in this text, is one way to confirm the quality characteristics of a final product—its software, its manufacturing process, and so on.

2. **Monitor quality characteristics.** Once the quality characteristics have been confirmed, programs must be in place to assure that products, manufacturing processes, test methods, and equipment routinely meet quality characteristics.

When validation is complete, monitoring and control programs must be initiated to ensure that the conditions of the validation are met routinely.

3. **Monitor for change and control change.** Change will occur. It is a basic principle of quality assurance, however, to establish systems that

   • Prevent unexpected change or minimize the likelihood of its occurrence,

   • Detect change when it occurs, and

   • Control change when it is necessary.

Observations of unexpected change to validated processes, methods, and equipment must be investigated. Planned changes to validated processes, methods, and equipment must be evaluated before change is implemented.

4. **Document!** There must be evidence that quality commitments have been fulfilled, and there must be a documented history of change.

The validation protocol must be written before validation begins. The validation data must support the commitments and meet the acceptance criteria of the validation protocol.

Quality Systems

In the complex regulatory environment of medical products manufacturing, the only way to meet the requirements of several regulatory agencies, international communities, and corporate commitments is to establish **systems** of compliance. Quality systems must honor the basic principles of quality assurance described above. In order to provide efficient and effective management of commitments, however, these systems must be custom designed for one's product, technology, manufacturing facility, and corporate culture. A good quality system will minimize redundancy, assure access to information, and integrate information from all disciplines and all levels of the organization.

A quality system also offers the advantage of flexibility. In an industry where standards change frequently, where new management can impose new directives, and where new products and new technologies evolve quickly, a rigorous yet flexible quality system provides the stability and assurance that can allow a corporation to respond proactively to its market and competition without risking product quality or patient safety.

Quality Manuals and Quality Plans

The quality system of a corporation is described in a *Quality Manual*. This term, which originated in the international community, refers to a document or a collection of documents that describes the corporate commitments to quality assurance. The *Quality Manual* references individual documents, such as departmental quality plans, that describe specific commitments and lead the reader, in turn, to more specific, directive documents such as standard operating procedures. Quality plans appropriate for a medical product manufacturer's *Quality Manual* include the following:

- Design development/preproduction quality assurance
- Manufacturing facility design, organization, and operation
- Validation
- Monitoring and control quality programs
- Documentation
- Change prevention, detection, and control
- Employee training
- Product-specific manufacturing
- Installation and servicing

The Commitment to Validate

Validation is not a one-time event. It is a quality assurance tool and, as such, it must be an ongoing commitment that is integral to every aspect of commercial product manufacturing. Given the potential complexity of the commitment, a systematic approach to validation is appropriate. Validation must confirm the quality of individual equipment systems, test methods, and software, as well as the quality of their interaction in the manufacturing process.

The commitments of validation must be communicated to both employees and regulators by describing how the commitments will be fulfilled in a manner appropriate to one's product, technology, manufacturing facility, and corporate philosophies. A Validation Master Plan or a Validation Quality Plan can serve this purpose; examples are presented in chapters 7 and 9.

This corporate systems approach to validation, involving written plans and programs, may seem absurd and unnecessary for a small device manufacturer with a single product. What can they do to comply with the *Code of Federal Regulations* and the *Medical Device Directives*? The answer: Ensure that the basic principles of quality assurance are honored in the work that is done. In this text we will present information about validation that should serve the needs of both the small, single-product manufacturer and the multiproduct, multinational organization.

Reference

Quality Management and Quality System Elements: Guidelines. 1987. ANSI/ASQC Q94-1987. Milwaukee: American Society for Quality Control.

Chapter 2

Validation

A History of Validation

Validation, along with Good Manufacturing Practices, was introduced into the pharmaceutical manufacturing industry in the mid-1970s in response to numerous problems with the sterility of large volume parenterals (LVPs). Prior to this time, validation had been applied only to analytical test methods in a laboratory setting. This new focus on sterilization validation, therefore, introduced validation into the production facility. By 1975 the validation of all sterilization processes was expected (i.e., steam sterilization, dry heat sterilization and depyrogenation, ethylene oxide sterilization, steam-in-place, filtration sterilization, and radiation sterilization).

By the late 1970s the expectation of validation included other critical activities associated with aseptic processing, such as media fills, environmental control, and sanitization. In addition and in response to numerous problems associated with water purification, water system validation became an expected practice. By 1983 validation was here to stay, and the *Guideline on General Principles of Process Validation* was first published.

Nonaseptic processes (such as tablet and capsule production) became candidates for validation, and the Pharmaceutical Manufacturers Association established the Computer System Validation Committee to address FDA concerns about computer systems used in products, product manufacturing, and storage and distribution systems.

Although the revised 1987 *Guideline on General Principles of Process Validation* included device manufacturers, the majority of the literature interpreting validation requirements came from the pharmaceutical industry (i.e., trade associations, trade journals, and the Center for Drugs and Biologics). This trend has continued and, as a result, validation has not been perceived by device manufacturers to be a high priority until lately.

Regulations, Guidelines, and Expectations

The passage of the Safe Medical Device Act of 1990, the new PMA initiatives compliance program of 1991, court cases in 1992, and the proposed revisions of Good Manufacturing Practices (21 CFR 820) have increased agency enforcement of validation for the device manufacturer.

Validation, however, is not new; the concepts of validation have been applied, successfully, for 15 years in drug and biologic manufacturing. Lessons have been learned. One lesson is that decisions must be made when designing and planning validation commitments. The concepts of validation are universal, and device manufacturers, given the scarcity of device-specific literature from the Center for Devices and Radiological Health, can learn from the experiences of the drug industry. This learning, however, must be applied appropriately to the device manufacturing environment. Each manufacturer must consider the information available from **all** sources when designing an effective compliance program.

Currently, the most informative FDA text on device validation is found in the fifth edition of the *Medical Device GMP Manual.* This manual also contains four other relevant documents:

1. "Guidelines on the General Principles of Process Validation"

2. "Application of the Medical Device GMPs to Computerized Devices and Manufacturing Processes"

3. "Preproduction Quality Assurance Planning: Recommendations for Medical Device Manufacturers"

4. "Guideline for the Manufacture of In Vitro Diagnostic Products"

When Is Validation Required?
When Is Validation Appropriate?

According to the proposed GMPs, one *must* validate "special processes." A special process is one in which the quality or the effectiveness of processing cannot be adequately tested or evaluated in the final product. This includes sterilizers, device software, and many device manufacturing processes.

There are other times when validation is appropriate. Consider validation for

- Utility systems, processing equipment, test equipment, software, or process whose failure could directly affect the safety of the product, patient, consumer, or user.

- Any event that requires routine, intensive monitoring and testing programs to confirm its quality and effectiveness. Validation can be used to eliminate or minimize routine testing commitments.

- Any equipment, processing, or software that is unique or custom designed. Unique systems do not benefit from widespread industry use and experience to support any expectation or history of consistent performance.

- Any equipment, processing, or software whose reliability or reproducibility is unknown or suspect. The validation process can offer the benefit of identifying highly variable components, subsystems, or equipment that can be upgraded or changed. Significant change, however, will necessitate another validation.

When in the Product Life Cycle to Validate?

Validation must occur when new products are brought to commercial production; validation should occur before new products are manufactured for human use.

So what does this mean? Clearly, a manufacturer does not want to commit to full-scale production and validation of a product before clinical trial testing in humans. So how does one proceed through product development and verification events, including clinical testing, and meet the expectations of the FDA for validation?

First consider the FDA's perspective: When a device manufacturer is given permission to market a device, this permission is sometimes granted based on data gathered in a clinical trial for PMA products and Class III 510ks. The quality of the clinical data is directly dependent on the quality of the product used; the quality of the product is directly dependent on the quality of the manufacturing process. If something changes in this relationship (the device, the device manufacturing process, or the clinical application), then the conclusions drawn from the relationship (approval to market) are suspect.

It is the responsibility of the manufacturer, therefore, to assure the FDA that this relationship has not been violated. If it is necessary to produce product for clinical evaluation in the development laboratory, then the manufacturer must be able to assure an investigator that the components, subassemblies, manufacturing process, and product consistently meet predetermined specifications by presenting documentation that demonstrates these facts. When product manufacturing is finally transferred to a commercial production environment, then the manufacturer must assure, through product processing validation, that the final product is equivalent to the product used in clinical testing.

Validation vs. Verification

Both verification and validation require that evidence be collected to demonstrate that specified requirements have been met by a process and/or a product. *Verification* is usually performed during product development to assure that the requirements for the product are met by the current version of the design, prototype, or product. *Validation* is a terminal event to product development and demonstrates that the commercial scale manufacturing process will, in fact, **consistently** produce a product that meets the predetermined specifications of the developed product.

There are fundamental differences between verification and validation. The primary difference is that validation demonstrates consistency. This means that one must demonstrate that specified requirements are met **multiple** times; at least three replicate events are usually sufficient. In addition, to demonstrate consistency, replicate runs must be identical. *Identical* means that processing parameters must fall within predetermined limits of acceptability. Processing parameters that must be controlled include lot size. This means that the validation of a manufacturing process should occur with the lot size that will be manufactured routinely, and consistency should be demonstrated with at least three commercial scale lots. Scale-up of a manufacturing process can be a significant change and may require revalidation.

Another aspect common to validation, but not to verification, is that the process, equipment, software, or method is challenged. This challenge consists of demonstrating that an acceptable outcome can be achieved when operating at processing limits and/or when operating at the extremes of capacity, volume, or load.

Fundamental Elements of Validation

Every validation event must

- Document the validation plan and procedures in controlled documents **before** validation begins;

- Establish acceptance criteria for the validation event **before** the validation begins (i.e., testing parameters, limits of acceptability, and methods of analysis for equipment performance, processing events, and the product of the processing event;

- Demonstrate that supporting equipment and equipment systems are calibrated and operate properly during validation events;

- Demonstrate that the **process** meets an established range of operation, for predetermined parameters, for multiple runs according to valid test procedures;

- Demonstrate that the **product** of the process or equipment system meets predetermined quality characteristics for multiple runs according to valid test procedures;

- Demonstrate the ruggedness of equipment or process performance by challenging the equipment or process at the limits of established operating conditions for multiple runs;

- Demonstrate the appropriateness, accuracy, precision, and so on of any analytical test method used to assess the performance, identity, strength, potency of chemical substances, components, equipment, processing, or product;

- Demonstrate the correlation and appropriateness of indicator testing that will be used to monitor the process or product during routine production; and

- Demonstrate that the validation event has been performed as planned and that the outcome of the event meets predetermined specifications and that the event has been documented, reviewed, and approved according to established procedures.

Validation Terminology and Definitions

The terminology of validation is very confusing. This confusion has resulted from an inconsistency of definition between the FDA, industry groups, and internationally. Although the definition of process validation, as it appears in the 1987 *Guideline on General Principles of Process Validation,* is generally accepted, the terminology beyond that is not.

For example, it is generally accepted that a validation event contains a subset of qualification events. An equipment system validation event would consist of an installation qualification (IQ), an operational qualification (OQ), and a performance qualification (PQ). The definition of these qualification events, however, varies from facility to facility.

Investigators have come to recognize this issue and, as a result, often ask for the corporate definitions of these terms before inspecting validation records. Clearly, what matters is that there is consistency of definition within a corporation and that the tasks commonly recognized as fundamental to IQ, OQ, and PQ evaluations are performed.

The calibration of equipment, measuring devices, and sensors, for example, is required during a validation event. Some companies choose to include this requirement in the installation qualification event while others include it in operational qualification. The location of the information does not matter as much as the commitment to perform calibration and the evidence that it has been done in a timely and appropriate manner.

Similarly, the word *validation* means different things to different people. When an investigator asks if a process has been validated, the response is usually "Yes." The investigator then asks to see what work has been performed to support this declaration and may see a variety of programs and commitments, ranging from a historical review of final product data to complete, prospective validation protocols and data packages. By viewing the evidence the inspector draws conclusions about the corporate commitments and definitions of validation.

Every corporation has its own definitions and approach to validation. If they are written down, an investigator will confirm that they were fulfilled by looking at the data and documentation. If they are not written down, then the investigator will discover them by talking to the employees. Whatever one's corporate definition and approach to validation, it is important that employees have a consistent understanding of this commitment and response to investigators.

How Much Testing Is Enough?

A complete validation of every utility system, every piece of processing or test equipment, every software program, and every manufacturing process would be a full-time commitment for the manufacturing staff. Not every system or every piece of equipment or every process requires the same level of evaluation. But what level of evaluation is appropriate? What are the options, and how does one make these decisions?

Utility systems validation (i.e., IQ, OQ, and PQ evaluations) is appropriate if the product of the system (water, air, steam, power) comes in direct contact with an invasive or implantable product. Validation is appropriate when the performance of the utility system or equipment directly affects product safety. In a steam-sterilized product, for example, both the sterilizer and the clean steam would require validation.

Similarly, if utility systems, processing equipment, or software has been designed in-house, or if vendor-supplied equipment is used in a manner other than that recommended by the vendor, validation may be required.

If validation is not appropriate, options for evaluation include performing only an IQ or an IQ/OQ. If the equipment is simple, routine preventive maintenance programs and routine calibration alone may be sufficient to establish the reliability and reproducibility of its performance.

Some equipment can be maintained and routinely calibrated to assure its reliable, reproducible performance. This equipment includes simple measuring devices such as calipers, balances, pH meters, conductivity meters, and pipettes.

The same concepts apply to manufacturing process validation decisions. Process validation may be appropriate when the product of the process is an invasive or implantable device; when inconsistent processing could directly affect the safety, performance, and quality of the final product; when the quality of the process cannot be detected or tested in final product; or when processing is unique. Similarly, as there are processes that require validation, some processes can be adequately controlled with the use of standards and positive and negative controls.

When these testing decisions are made, it may be useful to categorize the equipment into *levels of concern.* This categorization will be discussed throughout the text.

Approaches to Validation: Prospective, Retrospective, and Concurrent

Several approaches to validation are discussed in existing literature—prospective, retrospective, and concurrent validation. The simplest approach to validation is *prospective,* which means that **after** a product is developed, the product and its manufacturing process are validated **before** it is either introduced into the commercial market or used in humans.

Prospective validation, however, is not always possible. Given the new emphasis on process validation in the industry, many manufacturers are faced with validating products and processes that have been on the market for many years. Can this be done effectively? How does it differ from traditional, prospective validation events?

Retrospective validation means the validation of a process, a method, or equipment that has been in use for a long time or a product that has already been on the market. It can be effective only if both the processing events and the product have been monitored routinely for all important quality parameters, if there is an accurate and detailed history of change, and if the documentation to support processing, testing, and change is retrievable. In addition, one must be able to demonstrate that the processing occurred in a GMP environment. This means that the support

systems of monitoring and control, such as preventive maintenance programs, calibration programs, environmental monitoring
programs, electrostatic discharge programs, and employee training programs, were in effect and documented. Performing retrospective validation, as a result, is often a much more difficult and
intensive task than prospective validation.

Consider the advice to the FDA from Judge Wolin's interpretations of GMP issues contained in the Supreme Court's Ruling in
USA vs. Barr Laboratories:

> The court ruled that batches meeting the following criteria
> must be included in retrospective validation studies:
>
> 1. All batches made in the specified time period chosen
>   for study must be included unless the batch was made
>   from a non-process related error.
>
> 2. Only batches made in accord with the process evalu-
>   ated can be included.
>
> The number of retrospective batches chosen for the study
> must be greater than the number used for prospective vali-
> dation. Although the court set no exact number of batches
> to be chosen, guidelines have been established as follows:
>
> - Five batches is unacceptable and also six or more may not
>   be acceptable.
>
> - Because 10 percent batch failure is unacceptable, if one
>   batch fails, more than 10 batches are needed for the retro-
>   spective study.
>
> - Experts accept 20–30 batches.

When considering retrospective validation, review the product
description and its claims as described in the original 510k application or PMA. Determine, first of all, whether the product that is
manufactured is the same product or equivalent to product approved for market. If it is, then review the processing records and
ensure that processing has been consistent; that the product has
met specifications; that any deviations, complaints, or adverse
events associated with the product have been investigated; and
that the rationale for all change has been documented, evaluated
when appropriate, and responded to when there has been potential impact on product performance, patient, user, or consumer
safety.

Given the difficulties usually encountered in a retrospective validation, what might be a reasonable approach? Perhaps it will be a combination of some prospective validation studies combined with retrospective data review and new commitments to the collection of concurrent validation data (i.e., data collected during routine production of the product). Determine what is appropriate, reasonable, and scientifically rigorous; document the plan and perform the validation event. No matter the approach to validation, the validation must be planned and acceptance criteria must be determined before work begins.

References

Agalloco, J. 1993. The Validation Life Cycle. *Journal of Parenteral Science and Technology,* May–June:142–147.

Chapman, K. G. 1991. A History of Validation in the United States: Part I. *Pharmaceutical Technology,* October:82–96.

Chapman, K. G. 1991. A History of Validation in the United States: Part II. *Pharmaceutical Technology,* November:54–70.

Davis, R. 1993. Judge Wolins' Interpretations of GMP Issues Contained in the Court's Ruling in *USA vs. Barr Laboratories,* 2/4/93, presented at the 17th International GMP Conference, Athens, GA.

Nally, J., and R. Kieffer. 1993. The Future of Validation: From QC/QA to TQ. *Pharmaceutical Technology,* October:106–116.

Tetzlaff, R. F., R. E. Shepherd, and A. J. LeBlanc. 1993. The Validation Story: Perspectives on the Systematic GMP Inspection Approach and Validation Development. *Pharmaceutical Technology,* March:100–116.

Chapter 3

Validation of Equipment and Equipment Systems

Reliability of equipment operation and performance must be assured. This assurance supports the validation of products produced using the equipment or the processing facilitated by the equipment. Assurance can be achieved in many ways.

The impact of equipment performance on the quality of the product processed can range from incidental to significant. There should be a variety of programs to support the evaluation of equipment operation in a manner that is appropriate, reasonable, and yet scientifically rigorous. Typical programs in a manufacturing facility include preventive maintenance programs, calibration and metrology programs, equipment qualification programs, and equipment validation programs. In this chapter we will present the basic requirements of these quality programs and provide guidance on how to make appropriate and effective testing plans.

What Equipment Requires Validation?

The first requirement of planning an equipment validation program is to know what equipment you have in the facility and to understand its function in relation to the product manufacturing or product testing requirements. Make a list. Candidates for the list include

- Manufacturing equipment (e.g., filling machines, lyophilizers, sterilizers, curing ovens, coating machines, extruders, and packaging machines)

- Support processing equipment (e.g., dishwashers, plate washers, board washers, incubators, and ovens)

- Test equipment (e.g., circuit board analyzers, test stations, and tensile testers)

- Utility system equipment (e.g., water systems, compressed air systems, and clean rooms)

- Measuring equipment (e.g., balances, pH meters, pipettes, calipers, and oscilloscopes)

Equipment that would not be appropriate for the list includes office equipment (copy machines, mail room balances, etc.); and basic laboratory, production, maintenance, and material-handling equipment that have no measuring functions or calibration requirements (vortex, stir plates, etc.).

Categorize the list into three *levels of concern,* based on the amount of evaluation that will be appropriate to assure reliable performance (e.g., Categories I, II, and III, with Category III having the greatest level of concern). First, list the equipment and equipment systems whose reliability can be assured through calibration and preventive maintenance programs, and classify these items as the lowest level of concern—Category I Equipment. Examples would include simple measuring equipment such as thermometers, balances, calipers, or pipettes; other examples might include conductivity meters, oscilloscopes, and viscometers. This equipment should be included in preventive maintenance and calibration programs, as appropriate, and should have equipment identity numbers and either installation qualification forms or equipment cards on file in the Maintenance Department.

Next, list the equipment and equipment systems that might require validation (i.e., the equipment with the highest level of concern); classify these as Category III Equipment. Examples would include sterilizers that sterilize final product, utility systems that supply raw materials such as water, air, or steam to critical product processing events, custom-designed processing equipment, processing equipment that processes product in a manner that cannot be tested in final product, and test equipment that measures critical parameters of product safety or performance. Other examples might include, depending on the circumstance, curing ovens, circuit board assembly equipment, and packaging equipment.

Finally, look at what is left. This should be equipment and equipment systems whose quality of performance can be assured through qualification (i.e., installation and operational qualification events), as will be described below. This final list is categorized as Category II Equipment. This means either that qualification constitutes enough testing to assure reliability (e.g., a compressed air system that does not come in direct contact with final product), or it means that the most appropriate challenge to equipment performance will be evaluated in conjunction with a process validation event. These options will be described in greater detail later in this text.

Equipment Validation Format and Content: Category III Equipment

The format of an equipment validation event has evolved from the early validation work with sterilizers. Equipment validation, as a result, is most commonly performed as a three-phase process consisting of installation qualification (IQ), operational qualification (OQ), and performance qualification (PQ) events.

As mentioned above, every corporation has its own definitions for these phases of evaluation. In the context of this text and in our experience, our definitions follow.

Installation Qualification

The purpose of the installation qualification event is to document the installation of equipment in a manner that allows for the efficient implementation of calibration and preventive maintenance programs and facilitates effective control of change to the equipment, over time.

After the initial installation event, an IQ document begins to look like an equipment specification. It should describe all of the critical features of the equipment (i.e., any component or feature that, if changed, could seriously affect the operation, performance, or safety of the equipment or the product).

The following information is appropriate for an installation qualification document:

- "As-built" drawings of the equipment or system

- Equipment or system requirements

- A statement declaring the adequacy of the equipment for its intended use

- Equipment identity characteristics

- Utility requirements

- Safety features

- Reference to operator or maintenance manuals

- Reference to vendor support services or parts suppliers

The IQ document should be completed by and signed by either a member of the maintenance staff or the individual who will be responsible for the maintenance and performance of the equipment.

Because installation specifications are judged against purchasing specifications and existing facility requirements, IQ documents can be completed before the protocols for operational or performance qualifications are written. This is particularly useful when validating the start-up of a new facility, as many problems with equipment vendors can be solved while the validation protocols are being written.

Operational Qualification

The purpose of an operational qualification is to confirm that the equipment operates as expected under ideal conditions. Clearly, the IQ should be completed before an OQ begins to ensure that any deviations in operational expectations are not a result of improper installation.

The plan for an operational qualification must be written before the work begins, whether the OQ is a stand-alone assessment or part of a validation event. The plan must include what will be done, how it will be done, acceptance criteria, and information on how raw data is handled or processed.

Activities usually associated with operational qualification events include the following:

- Calibration of sensors or measuring devices on the equipment or on test equipment used for this assessment

- Qualification of support processing such as equipment cleaning, disinfection, passivation, or sterilization

- Qualification of monitoring or controlling software

- Qualification or validation of the test methods used to assess performance

- A systematic demonstration of equipment electromechanical features and functions

- A demonstration of cycle performance, when appropriate, including the performance of programmed logic controllers or software programs

- A demonstration of process uniformity or consistency (e.g., heat distribution in an oven, fill volume uniformity on a filling machine, or moisture level uniformity in a lyophilizer)

- A demonstration of safety features and reset procedures after likely events such as a power failure

The acceptance criteria for an operational qualification event must assure that **both** the equipment processing parameters and the product of the processing event meet specifications.

During the writing of an operational qualification for a new equipment system, one learns about the equipment from vendor manuals, "as-built" drawings, and any historical experience with the equipment. With this knowledge one develops a validation or qualification plan to confirm that the equipment operates as expected.

This plan, however, must be supported by standard operating procedures on topics such as operating, cleaning, assembling, and calibrating the equipment, and performing routine maintenance on it. These procedures should be written and approved before the OQ begins. In addition, schedules for preventive maintenance (PM) and calibration should be determined and incorporated into existing programs for PM and calibration.

An operational qualification event is complete when the work directed by the protocol is complete and acceptable, when the supporting SOPs are written and approved, and when the routine commitments to equipment maintenance and calibration have been made.

Performance Qualification

The performance qualification event is the heart of validation. The performance qualification must confirm, under routine **and challenged** conditions of operation, that the equipment continues to operate as expected and that the outcome of processing is acceptable. This must be demonstrated repeatedly, which usually means a minimum of three consecutive successful runs.

Challenging the equipment to confirm its operation within the established limits of operation is a fundamental requirement of a performance qualification event. One should demonstrate reliable performance at the limits of acceptable operating conditions. This does not mean an endless number of demonstration runs with each parameter pushed to a minimum or maximum limit; it means that one should adopt a reasonable approach to the performance evaluation.

For example, if you are validating a heat sealing unit with parameters for temperature, pressure, and dwell time, it is not necessary to demonstrate the effect of the highest acceptable temperature, then the lowest temperature, highest pressure, and so on. It would be reasonable, however, to demonstrate the two extremes of operation that would most likely result in a poor seal. The first set of conditions would be the highest acceptable temperature, the highest acceptable pressure, and the longest acceptable dwell time; these conditions might result in a cut seal. The second set of conditions (i.e., lowest temperature, lowest pressure, and shortest dwell time) might result in an incomplete seal. If one can confirm that in each case the seals are acceptable, then when the equipment performs within those operating boundaries routinely, the sealing event could be judged as acceptable.

The performance qualification event should also confirm the appropriateness of the indicator monitoring or testing that will be used routinely to judge the performance of the equipment. If, for example, one plans to use a circular recording chart to routinely monitor the acceptability of an oven cycle, then one must confirm, during the PQ, that the circular chart correlates to established criteria for heat distribution.

Equipment vs. Equipment Systems

The evaluation of equipment performance must be considered in the context of how that equipment functions in use. Some pieces of equipment, like curing ovens, function independently from other processing equipment and are best evaluated as such. For utility systems and some processing and test equipment, however, where several equipment components interact to process a product, evaluation must assess the performance of the system, not simply the equipment. There are many equipment systems, including compressed air systems, water systems, clean rooms, and HPLC systems.

In order to distinguish between a piece of equipment and an equipment system, consider the product of the system. For example, a purified water system consists of softeners, carbon beds, ion exchange resin beds, filters, UV lights, a storage tank, a recirculating pump, and distribution piping. Since water is not removed from the system for use until it has been completely processed, the system should be evaluated as a whole. This means that it would be inappropriate to validate the softeners and then validate the resin beds and then the UV lights, and so on. It might be appropriate, however, to perform an installation and operational qualification on system components and then a performance qualification on the system as a whole.

This component qualification approach to validation is useful because it can minimize testing when changes occur in the system. When a water system fails because the recirculating pump requires replacement, for example, a full revalidation might be required. If the original evaluation was designed to qualify individual components of the system before validation of the entire system, however, it may be possible to evaluate the pump as a separate component and then run an abbreviated PQ on the entire water system.

New or Existing Systems

Validation may be appropriate when new equipment is installed, when existing equipment is used for new processing events, or when regulatory pressures suggest that it is appropriate to validate an existing, in-use system. The design of the validation protocol must consider the circumstances of the validation requirement.

Existing systems may have historical data that can be used to determine appropriate testing parameters and limits. New systems, however, may require use before appropriate limits can be set. There are two ways to achieve this: Either pick a reasonable but wide range of limits for test parameters and tighten these limits as appropriate over time, or conduct development studies on the equipment until its performance parameters and limits are understood sufficiently to design a validation protocol.

Test Equipment Evaluations

Validation and qualification requirements apply to test equipment as well as to manufacturing equipment. The commitments to test equipment qualification should be categorized using the same guidelines as described above (i.e., the accuracy and precision of Category I Equipment is assured through calibration and the use of standards, while Category III Equipment would require a full validation).

The Commitments of Routine Maintenance, Calibration, and Change Control

Qualification and validation events confirm that equipment operates as expected within an established range of operational parameters. To assure that the equipment performance matches the conditions of the qualification or validation over time, however, one must develop either monitoring and control programs or indicator testing programs to confirm that the conditions of the validation are routinely met.

The monitoring and control programs for equipment and equipment systems are preventive maintenance programs, calibration programs, and equipment change control programs. The first two programs are commonplace in most of the industry; the equipment change control program, however, can often be overlooked.

The changes that occur to equipment or equipment systems over time must be documented. A mechanic, for example, should not be able to change the seal in a recirculating pump of a validated equipment system without the notification or approval of quality assurance or the validation group. Similarly, a production technician should not be able to change the point-of-use sterilizing filter on a compressed air system without notifying QA.

These notifications can occur through the use of equipment work orders that simply record the occurrence of an event. These notification documents allow QA and/or the validation group to decide if the validation has been affected and whether additional testing or revalidation is appropriate. Without this documentation of change, however, equipment and equipment systems can operate in violation of their validation.

Chapter Appendix:
Validation of the Superior Autoclave for the Sterilization of Product XYZ—An Example

1.0 Purpose

This protocol describes the tasks required to demonstrate the ability of the superior autoclave to effectively, reliably, and consistently sterilize product XYZ.

2.0 Scope

This protocol applies to the superior autoclave used in manufacturing, equipment #23-A-234.

3.0 Responsibility

The tasks outlined in this protocol are directed by the validation specialist. Maintenance, Manufacturing, Quality Control, and Quality Assurance all participate in the evaluation and testing phases, as appropriate.

4.0 Protocol

4.1 Installation Qualification

The IQ will be completed according to SOP 123 or the existing IQ document will be reviewed by Maintenance and signed off as acceptable before proceeding to the operational qualification.

4.2 Operational Qualification

4.2.1. Preliminary Operations

4.2.1.1 Calibrate thermocouples and RTDs according to SOP 222. Must meet criteria of ±0.2°C.

4.2.1.2 Calibrate timing devices according to SOP 333. Must meet criteria of ±30 seconds.

4.2.1.3 Calibrate pressure gauges and pressure recording devices according to SOP 444. Must meet criteria of ±0.5 psig.

4.2.1.4 Calibrate temperature recording device according to SOP 555. Must meet criteria of ±1°C.

4.2.2 Heat Distribution/Empty Chamber

4.2.2.1 Placement of TCs and RTDs

Describe the exact placement of TCs and RTDs in this protocol. When performing this protocol, provide a diagram of the chamber with locations and TC numbers and RTD numbers indicated on the diagram. Place a TC in the drain!

4.2.2.2 Cycle Settings

Describe the cycle parameter settings (time, temperature, pressure, prevac, cooling, etc.) that will be used for this heat distribution study.

4.2.2.3 Cycle Data Collection Requirements

Describe the process of running the autoclave and what documentation is required (i.e., use of logbooks, record of cycle number, chart recordings, etc.). Refer to the SOP "Operation of the Autoclave," if one exists.

4.2.2.4 Heat Distribution Cycle Acceptance Criteria

Example Criteria:

- There are three consecutive heat distribution cycles.

- All thermocouples and RTDs are recording throughout at least two cycles; diagrams of TC and RTD placement are available for each cycle.

- All RTD and TC temperature recordings must be 121.6°C ±0.5°C for 30 minutes ±3 minutes (if a 30-minute cycle was set); documentation is available to support these observations.

- Pressure recording devices must meet 14.7 psig ±0.5 psig for 30 minutes ±3 minutes; documentation is available to support these observations.

- Three consecutive cycles must meet the above criteria before proceeding.

4.2.2.5 Identification of Cold Spots

Describe how the data will be analyzed to determine the cold spot in the chamber.

4.2.3   Heat Distribution/Loaded Chamber

It is common practice to perform a heat distribution on a loaded chamber of materials, such as a full load of product or placebo, just to see if the cold spot changes. This eliminates any surprises that may occur when heat penetration studies begin. Usually one run is sufficient for this evaluation. Note: If placebo or product is used, ensure that it is processed in a manner identical to that used routinely.

4.2.4   Cold Spot Determination

Describe the analysis of all data from this study and how it is used to document the uniformity of chamber conditions and the identification of the chamber cold spot.

4.3   Performance Qualification/Heat Penetration Studies

4.3.1   Preliminary Operations

4.3.1.1 Ensure that the biological indicators (*Bacillus stearothermophilus* PN 1234) meet specifications.

4.3.1.2 Ensure that the heat distribution studies have been approved by the validation committee.

4.3.1.3 Ensure that the cold spot, determined from the heat distribution studies, is monitored by a RTD.

4.3.1.4 When using materials that will routinely be washed and/or processed before exposure to steam sterilization, ensure that these materials have been processed before they are used in these studies.

4.3.2   Loading Configurations, Cycle Parameters, and Acceptance Criteria for Individual Heat Penetration Studies

4.3.2.1 Materials to Be Sterilized

List the materials to be sterilized and for each material load provide the following information:

- Loading configurations

- Location of thermocouples, RTDs, and biological indicators

- Cycle settings

- Acceptance criteria (e.g., cycle parameter acceptance criteria; TC/RTD acceptance criteria; biological indicator tests and acceptance criteria; number of consecutive, successful cycles required; load configuration requirements [min/max]; and a commitment that all raw data collection is complete and available for review)

4.3.3 Final Operations

When all studies are complete, calibrate thermocouples according to SOP 222; they must meet criteria of ±0.2°C.

4.3.4 Acceptance Criteria for Heat Penetration Studies

4.3.4.1 All available data from TCs and RTDs meet the following time/temperature requirements:

- 121.6°C ±0.5°C

- 30 minutes ±1 minute

- The raw data records are available to support these observations.

4.3.4.2 Pressure recording sensors meet the following criteria:

- 14.7 psig ±0.5 psig for 27–33 minutes

- The raw data records are available to support these observations.

4.3.4.3 The biological indicator in the cold spot has been tested according to SOP 1234 and is sterile.

4.3.4.4 All other available biological indicators have been tested according to SOP 1234 and are sterile.

4.3.4.5 This acceptance criteria must be met for three consecutive loads of each type of material

> processed. (Indicate three maximum and three minimum loads, if appropriate.)

5.0 Acceptance Criteria for Validation

- The guidelines and commitments in this protocol have been followed, met, and documented.

- The IQ, OQ, and PQ acceptance criteria have been met and documented.

- All raw data records are complete and available for review.

6.0 Documentation Requirements

The data from this validation is assembled by the validation specialist for review by the validation committee. When reviewed and found to be acceptable, the committee issues a validation certificate. This certificate is posted on or near the autoclave and declares an expiration date for the unit. The recommended expiration date is 1 year from the completion of the validation.

Validation data files/notebooks are kept in Documentation.

The recording charts that are generated from these validation cycles can be used to establish master charts for use by Production and QC personnel. SOPs, batch records, and preclearance procedures that cite these sterilization cycles should be reviewed and updated as appropriate as a result of this validation event.

References

Carleton, F. J., and J. P. Agalloco, eds. 1986. *Validation of Aseptic Pharmaceutical Processes.* New York: Marcel Dekker.

DeSain, C. V. 1993. *Drug, Device and Diagnostic Manufacturing: The Ultimate Resource Handbook.* 2nd ed. Buffalo Grove, IL: Interpharm Press.

Henke, C., and R. Reich. 1992. The Current Status of Microbial-Barrier Testing of Medical Device Packaging. *Medical Device and Diagnostic Industry,* August:46–94.

Hudson, B. J., and L. Simmons. 1992. Streamlining Package-Seal Validation. *Medical Device and Diagnostic Industry,* October: 49–52, 89.

Packaging for Terminally Sterilized Health Care Products: Final Product Package. ISO 11607-3.

Packaging for Terminally Sterilized Health Care Products: Forming and Sealing. ISO 11607-2.

Packaging for Terminally Sterilized Health Care Products: Packaging Materials. ISO 11607-1.

Spitzley, J. 1991. A Preview of the HIMA Sterile Packaging Guidance Document. *Medical Device and Diagnostic Industry,* December:59–61.

Stellon, R. C. 1986. Sterile Packaging Validation. *Medical Device and Diagnostic Industry,* October:42–46.

Sterilization of Health Care Products: Requirements for Validation and Routine Control: Industrial Moist Heat Sterilization. ISO 11134.

Sterilization of Health Care Products: Requirements for Validation and Routine Control: Gamma and Electron Beam Radiation Sterilization. ISO 11137-2.

Validation and Routine Control of EtO Sterilization. ISO 11135.2.

Validation of Dry Heat Processes Used for Sterilization and Depyrogenation. Technical Bulletin No. 3. Bethesda, MD: Parenteral Drug Association.

Chapter 4

Test Method Validation

The safety and performance characteristics of products, processes, and equipment must be judged by methods that are reliable. Test method validation is a fundamental building block of any quality assurance system and should be one of the first validation programs initiated during the development of a new product or the start-up of a new facility.

Historically, test method validation has been the responsibility of the research and development laboratory. Test methods for drug and biologic products have been developed and then submitted along with samples of the product to the FDA for approval. The FDA (Center for Drug Evaluation and Research) confirms the suitability and reliability of the test methods. If the methods are unacceptable, the product application is not approved. As a result, test method validation has been focused primarily on product testing (i.e., tests that determine product safety, performance, uniformity, stability, or reliability); the need to validate raw material or in-process test methods has been minimized.

Although this history has resulted in little guidance from the FDA on either the validation of standard methods or the application of GMPs in a laboratory setting, the tide is turning. The requirements for method validation now extend beyond product-specific assays and test methods to include raw material, equipment, environmental monitoring, and process-intermediate test methods. This means that some tests performed routinely in quality control or in production may require validation.

One reason that the traditional approach to test method validation is changing is the result of recent FDA inspections of quality control and research laboratories. Inspectors have found significant GMP violations in these laboratories; these violations call into question the quality of data generated by the laboratory. Agency inspection experience resulted in the publication of the *Guide to the Inspections of Pharmaceutical Quality Control Laboratories* in July 1993. In addition, inspectors now visit test laboratories during routine inspections and look for GMP violations.

So how does one prepare for test method validation? Which methods require validation and which do not? How are these decisions made? How are methods validated in a manner that would be acceptable to an FDA reviewer or an FDA inspector?

Test Method Categorization

First, make a list of all test methods currently used to assess quality parameters for products, raw materials, utility systems, environmental systems, equipment performance, software, and so on. List the method, the purpose of the method, and what types of products or items are currently tested by this method.

The rigor of a test method validation should correlate with what is tested, the purpose of the test, and the complexity or uniqueness of the test method. Group the methods into three categories. Category I Methods include tests that are compendium tests or well-accepted methods whose reliability can be easily assured with standards, controls, and calibration commitments. Tests in Category I would include Lowry protein assays, pH measurements, caliper measurements, viscosity, and melting points.

Category III Methods require full validation. This category would be appropriate for any method whose result directly affects the safety of a product, any method that is unique or custom designed, and any method whose reliability is unknown or suspect. Tests in Category III would include pyrogen tests; sterility tests; unique performance or potency tests; unique flex, torque, and stiffness test methods; and sterile barrier challenge tests.

Category II Methods include everything else. The proper evaluation of these methods might include equipment qualification events and some demonstration of accuracy, precision, or ruggedness, but not a full demonstration of reliability or challenge.

With these categories determined, the rigor of testing that is appropriate for individual tests can be determined. Consider what is being tested, the testing parameter evaluated, and the suitability of the test to provide appropriate and reliable information.

What Is Being Tested?

- Is this final product? Is the product implantable, invasive, or in vitro?

- Is this a critical component or subassembly of the final product?

- Could variation in this item adversely affect the safety or performance of the product?

What Is the Testing Parameter?

- Does the test determine the safety of a product (e.g., contaminant testing, impurity testing, hazards testing)?

- Does the test determine product performance where performance failure could adversely affect the patient?

What Is the Suitability and Reliability of the Test?

- Why is this the best test for measuring this parameter?

- Is the test unique or custom designed? Is there historical data on its performance to support its accuracy and precision?

- Is the test an accepted USP or compendium test?

- Is there another analysis, performed routinely on the product, that confirms the results of this test?

Test Method Validation Plan: Format and Content

Test method validation protocols should follow the basic format provided in USP 23 with the addition of GMP requirements and concerns. Consider the following sections when formatting your test method validation plan.

- **Method principles:** Describe the general principles at work in the analysis. If appropriate, refer to the method development report.

- **Method suitability:** Describe why this method is suitable for determining the given parameter; declare any known limitations to its suitability.

- **Method categorization:** Declare the appropriate category of evaluation, as described above.

- **Raw material and component controls:** List the materials required to perform the method, including standards and controls, and indicate their required quality characteristics.

- **Sample acceptance criteria:** Indicate any sample handling requirements or sample suitability limitations.

- **Equipment controls and calibration:** List the equipment required for the analysis and any calibration requirements.

- **Technician training:** If specific training is required for the performance of the test method, indicate this.

- **Test method SOP:** The test method must be written and followed in order to perform the validation event. The procedure should describe how to do the method in a step-by-step manner; it should give exact measurements and provide examples of how to make calculations or how to handle data.

- **Evaluation:** The precision of the method should be confirmed under ideal conditions. If appropriate, accuracy should also be confirmed. These analyses should be performed with sufficient replicates to provide some statistical significance to the method. These accuracy and precision values will be used as a standard against which the ruggedness of the method will be evaluated when challenged later.

    When appropriate, the limits of detection, the limits of quantitation, selectivity, specificity, interferences, linearity, and range should also be confirmed. If the analysis is performed in conjunction with another test for the same parameter or if it is replacing an existing test, then correlation should be determined between the tests.

    Method validation is an opportunity to confirm the ruggedness of the test. Demonstrate that the precision and accuracy limits are met with different technicians, different lots of raw materials or components, different vendors, variable sampling storage times, variable sample methods, variable test equipment, and so on.

Finally, ensure the correlation of indicator testing (i.e., those tests, controls, or standards that will be used routinely to assess the validity of the method) with the validation data.

- **Acceptance criteria:** Describe what results are considered acceptable (e.g., precision and accuracy limits, limits of detection and quantitation, types of samples, storage times, etc.). Also describe data handling techniques and requirements.

- **Documentation requirements:** Describe how the data will be recorded and filed.

Routine Monitoring of a Validated Test Method

Every time a method is performed, there should be standards, controls, relative standard deviation limits, correlation coefficients, or some indicator test to ensure that the conditions of the qualification or validation continue to be met. These requirements should be incorporated into the test method SOP.

A test method generally follows an SOP, and the data generated from the analysis is recorded on a device manufacturing record, on a data collection form, or in a logbook. These data records should always indicate the method used to perform the work; such references should include the document number and its revision level.

Raw data should be stored in a location that best facilitates its appropriate use. If the data concerns the performance of manufacturing equipment, for example, it might be appropriate to collect this data in an equipment logbook. If the data is specific to a lot of product, then it is appropriate for the data to be recorded on the device manufacturing record.

When it is useful to have two sets of data on file, for example, one chronological and one by product, then ensure that the original data is always stored in the same place. Do not mix original data with copies of original data. An FDA inspector will always want to see the original data.

Out-of-Specification Results

Given that a common reason for enforcement action against a manufacturer is inadequate response to out-of-specification (OOS) results, we will review the issues and concerns as they apply to validation.

You must not ignore or discount unacceptable results without adequate rationale or scientific justification; this rationale must be documented. Out-of-specification results must be investigated; investigations must be appropriate, competent, timely, and complete.

An OOS result does not automatically result in the rejection of product or the failure of the validation event, but that possibility must be considered. There are initially several reasons that a test method produces an OOS result (e.g., inappropriate equipment performance, poor sampling technique, an adulterated sample, a mistake by the technician). The response to the event, however, must be rational (i.e., resampling and retesting must not be an automatic response to the wrong result).

All OOS results that occur during a validation event must be investigated. Every investigation should be documented.

Training of Technicians

The analyst is the first line of defense against the occurrence of OOS results. Analysts must be properly trained to perform the test methods, and they must be observant of all associated equipment, environmental, and sample parameters that could affect the quality or accuracy of the results. Technicians must be trained to perform test methods before they validate these methods.

The FDA's Paul Vogel suggests the following basic principles be applied by analysts in the laboratory:

- The analyst must not deviate from the validated methods or standard procedures.

- Deviations must be documented, explained, and evaluated by the supervisor.

- Equipment and instruments must not be used unless they are known to be properly maintained and calibrated.

- The analyst must document procedural glitches, such as spilling samples or other problems.

- The analyst should not knowingly continue a procedure that she/he expects to invalidate later due to an appropriate, assignable cause.

- Analysts must be encouraged to say, "I might have made a mistake."

References

Analytical Validation. 1990. *Rules Governing Medicinal Production in the European Community,* Volume IIIA, Brussels - Luxembourg: Commission of the European Communities, July:1–16.

Analysts Can Forestall OOS Results. 1993. *The Gold Sheet,* October:5.

DeSain, C. V. 1992. Master Method Validation Protocols. *BioPharm,* June:30–34.

DeSain, C. V. 1993. *Documentation Basics That Support Good Manufacturing Practices.* Cleveland: Advanstar Communications, Cleveland.

FDA Compliance Official Vogel Discusses Implications of Barr Decision. 1993. *The Gold Sheet,* October:9–12.

Finkelson, M. J. 1986. Validation of Analytical Methods by FDA Laboratories II. *Pharmaceutical Technology,* March:75, 78, 80–84.

Guerra, J. 1986. Validation of Analytical Methods by FDA Laboratories I. *Pharmaceutical Technology,* March:74, 76, 78.

Morris, J. M. 1989. US and EEC Requirements for Documenting Process and Methods Validation. *Drug Information Journal,* Vol. 23:453–461.

Validation of Compendial Methods. 1995. *U.S. Pharmacopeia 23,* Chapter 1225.

Chapter 5

Validation of Automated Equipment Systems and Software

When someone mentions software validation, two distinct types come to mind: validation of computerized products and validation of automated manufacturing or test equipment. Within each type there are varying levels of appropriate concern and evaluation, but it is important to start with this general division.

This chapter will discuss the validation of automated systems. An automated system is a collection of multiple equipment units with one or more microprocessors and associated hardware and software. The system controls, monitors, or reports a specific set of sequential activities without human intervention. Examples of automated systems include sterilizers, computerized drill presses, lathes, punches, test stations, HPLC systems, clean-in-place units, and inventory management systems.

Clearly, the problems resulting from the faulty performance of automated systems could have a significant affect on patient safety and product performance. As a result, validations should be designed to demonstrate that the systems are free of error and reliable. This means that the data generated from the system or process are accurate and reliable.

Automated System Inventory

The first priority for the qualification or validation of automated, computerized systems is to have an inventory of the system and its components. Make a list of all automated systems that support Good Manufacturing Practices. The FDA requires a manufacturer to demonstrate control of software systems involved in manufacturing, testing, storing, and distributing product. Associate and identify the items on the list with the automated processes that they report, monitor, and/or control. List the physical location of the system and the name of the software used in the system, if available. In addition, if the equipment in the facility has been assigned equipment numbers, include those on the list to distinguish between identical pieces of equipment.

Depending on the scope of work at your facility, you may also want to list data processing programs that handle clinical data or laboratory data. Similarly, consider the programmable personal calculators or computers used to calculate production or laboratory data. These personal tools are often the source of error.

Categorization of Concern

When the list of automated systems has been compiled, begin to make decisions about the rigor of evaluation, qualification, or validation that would be appropriate to each system. As with the other validation decisions discussed in this book, it is appropriate to segregate the list into three categories of concern.

Category I Systems are those that do not directly affect the safety, uniformity, or performance of the product or the manufacturing process or those processes whose reliability is easily confirmed with standards and calibration.

Category III Systems directly affect product safety and/or are custom designed and/or their reliability is unknown or suspect. The most obvious example of a process requiring a Category III validation commitment is a sterilizer that sterilizes final product. Failure of an automated sterilization cycle would not necessarily be detected by final product testing and could have a serious affect on patient safety.

Category II Systems are those that affect the performance of the product or its uniformity but do not require full validation. An example of a process appropriate for Category II qualification studies would be a drying oven controlled by a programmed logic controller. It would be appropriate to demonstrate that the various programmed cycles perform as intended (i.e., to perform an operational qualification), but it may not be appropriate to challenge the performance of the software separate from equipment performance qualification.

In addition to the system concerns influencing the categorization, one must consider the origin of the software. Is this an off-the-shelf program, a user-modified program, or a program written in-house? A program that has been used by hundreds of manufacturers in the industry without complaint will require a less rigorous evaluation than a custom-designed program.

Validation Options for Automated Systems

Develop options for validation (i.e., the tools you can use to evaluate and confirm the reliability of software performance). Options can include the following:

- Gathering vendor and user information on the system's performance and reliability. Clearly, if the system has been used by thousands of users and has a reputation for reliability, then the user must demonstrate that this reliability continues.

- Performing structural tests (e.g., source code or pathway analysis).

- Performing functional tests (e.g., side-by-side testing and test sets). Design test sets to find errors in the programming, not simply to demonstrate reliability. If the consistent operation of different modules of the system is demonstrated, also demonstrate the reliability of the integration of information from these modules. The reliability of the parts does not necessarily equal the reliability of the whole.

Can Software Validation Be Performed in Conjunction with Equipment System Validation?

When software is used to monitor, control, and report the performance of equipment systems, it becomes difficult to draw the line between the validation of the equipment and the validation of the software. There are, however, a few points to consider in this decision making.

Validation of a software-driven system should focus primarily on validating the product of the system. In the case of a water treatment system, the product is water; in the case of an analytical test, the product may be data; in the case of a product manufacturing event, the product may be a subassembly. The validation that matters, ultimately, is the validation of the overall system. To achieve this validation in a logical manner, however, one must qualify certain components and subprocessing BEFORE the system is validated. Software qualification can be one of these requirements.

How does software qualification differ from software validation? Software qualification requires documentation of the installation of the unit. In a software-driven, computerized equipment system the installation of the computer hardware is documented just like other system equipment components in an IQ document. Similarly, the software is identified and controlled as discussed above.

When the IQ is complete, an OQ event can be performed. The software can be exercised to demonstrate that it can perform the functions appropriately and in proper sequence without any demonstration of ruggedness or challenge. Again, in a complex system it is often difficult to separate software OQ from equipment or process OQ. They need not be separated as long as their successful operation is sufficiently demonstrated.

When qualification is complete, the system can be operated as a whole to demonstrate the consistency of the overall processing event and the consistent quality characteristics of the final product. In this way the performance of the software is demonstrated and challenged along with the performance of the equipment systems it supports and the product processed.

Simple Equipment Systems Should Require Simple Evaluation

Evaluate the performance of the system in a manner that is rigorous but also appropriate and reasonable to its application. According to the FDA, validation is appropriate for "special processes" (i.e., those processes whose outcome cannot be adequately tested in the final product).

In an automated drill press, for example, whose size, angle, and configuration of the holes after the drilling event can be measured, validation would not be necessary. It might be appropriate, however, to ensure the accuracy of the drill bits by calibration and to institute a preventive maintenance program for the drill press and the bits.

For a drying oven that has no test to measure the effectiveness of the drying event on the product, then validation might be appropriate. Validation would require equipment IQ and OQ events that include the calibration of timers, thermometers, thermocouples, and RTDs, as well as a demonstration of all electromechanical features of the cycles under ideal conditions and a demonstration of heat distribution in an empty oven chamber. The PQ would require a demonstration of the uniformity of heat distribution in a fully loaded oven and some testing to demonstrate that the product processed by this oven cycle is acceptably dry.

A Note About Manual Systems

If the majority of work is done manually, then equipment validation is essentially eliminated as a validation commitment. One must always demonstrate the consistency of processing, however, and determine the best way to design this demonstration.

The consistency and success of manual processing depends directly on the quality of the instructions and the training and expertise of the technicians performing the work. Making an equation between the instructions in a manual operation and software in an automated operation requires a commitment to strict control of the instructions. Procedures, batch records, and history records must be followed routinely, and there must be evidence to support their use and control.

The Validation Protocol

The approach to validation will vary with the complexity of the computerized system. What follows is simply an outline of points to consider when designing the format of a validation protocol for a computerized, automated process.

1.0 Introduction

The commitment to validation and the history of the processing event and its evaluation and validation is presented here.

2.0 System Description: Installation Qualification

2.1 The Processing Event

Describe what this system does and what is automated (i.e., What is the product or outcome of the automated processing event? What are the raw materials of the process? What are the intermediate steps, [if appropriate]?).

If there is an SOP, a device manufacturing record, or a batch record associated with this event, cite the document number and the revision level of the document that will be used during this validation event.

2.2 Equipment Components

List and/or describe the equipment and hardware components. Be specific. This section is equivalent to the IQ section of an equipment validation protocol. Include the location of this equipment in the facility. Include a list of the input and output devices and the input and output requirements for each device. Consider listing transducers, sensors, valves, actuators, thermocouples, RTDs, microswitches, weight cells, and level controllers. Describe interfaces and communication options available for computerized systems.

2.3 Software Components

List the software and its revision level. If appropriate, provide the program structure tree/algorithm and/or code, and/or describe the cycles. If there is not a separate software specification, describe the software database management system, networking capabilities, and other requirements.

2.4 System Limitations

Point 2.1 described what the system will do. Now is the opportunity to describe what it will **not** do. If there are limitations on processing as a result of sample types or scheduling or equipment capacities, declare them here.

2.5 System Safety and Security Features

Describe what is available.

3.0 Demonstration of System Performance: Operational Qualification

In this section describe how the performance of the software will be demonstrated. If this performance is demonstrated in conjunction with a processing event, ensure that sensors are calibrated prior to this event. Demonstrate each line of programmed function; demonstrate safety and security features; demonstrate backup and recovery; demonstrate that users are properly trained; demonstrate the effects of a power failure. Demonstrate that data from the system is properly archived and is retrievable.

Test sets can be designed to demonstrate proper performance. If a given test set is to be used routinely during production, ensure that this test set is run during the validation event to demonstrate its correlation to other data. For complex systems consider modular testing; ensure, however, that the system is tested as a whole after modular testing.

Declare how the data generated from this OQ event will be processed and the acceptance criteria for these OQ events.

4.0 Performance Qualification

As mentioned above, the qualification of a computerized processing event may end with the IQ and OQ. In this case the performance of the software will be challenged eventually by processing actual product. When this demonstration is completed, there must be evidence of reproducibility, consistency, or uniformity and ruggedness of the process and the product.

5.0 Validation Acceptance Criteria

Declare the overall acceptance criteria for the validation event.

6.0 Documentation Requirements

Describe the review and approval requirements for the validation.

System Support After Validation

After the validation is complete, there must be systems in place to detect change to the hardware, the software, and the processing event. Similarly, there must be change review and evaluation programs or procedures. Few changes to a computerized system affect a single aspect of the system. Changes to computerized systems, therefore, require a thorough understanding of the system and the consequences of change. This can only be achieved with a multidisciplinary review of change.

When changes occur to computerized, automated processes, there should be several options for the evaluation of change. These options should vary from simple on-line verification activities to off-line development/verification and revalidation. Change is discussed in chapter 11; revalidation is discussed in chapter 12.

Finally, the performance of computerized, automated systems should be audited routinely by QA to ensure that they continue to perform as intended.

Chapter Appendix:
GMP Points to Consider

Software Identification and Control

Make a list of the software used in the facility. This list should be used to assign part numbers and revision level numbers to the software. If convenient, use the current part numbering system for these number assignments by designating a separate series of numbers for software.

Software is a set of important, detailed instructions that must be used routinely to perform tasks. As such, software is like a standard operating procedure, a device manufacturing record, or a batch record and should be controlled appropriately and similarly.

With these number assignments, label all the original disks with their identification numbers and revision level, and then file them in a secure location in QA or Documentation. Make working copies for use on the manufacturing floor. To assist in the identification of master copies versus working copies, use distinct and different colored labels for these disks.

The filing system for software should also contain a specification for that software describing its attributes and a software history log to record revision level changes, the date of change, and a brief description of the change. In addition, the distribution of the software should be controlled and documented in a distribution log.

Some software, however, is configurable, but cannot be removed from the system for physical identification and filing. Such software programs should still be assigned identification and revision level numbers. Instead of filing the disk, however, print out the configurable program, review it, and file it in the documentation files. This master copy can be compared with the current program operating in the unit at any time to detect change. When a new configuration is entered, a new hard copy is generated and a new revision level assigned.

When all the software has been identified, label the associated hardware with the software identification and revision level approved for use with that unit.

Hardware Configuration Management

Computerized hardware systems should also be identified and controlled. If the facility has already instituted an equipment identification numbering system, use it. If this system also allows for the identification of equipment systems, then it will work well for computerized equipment; if not, try to extend the existing system to accommodate these requirements.

An equipment system is a collection of interacting equipment components. A compressed air system, for example, contains a compressor, a storage tank, a drying unit, filters, distribution piping, point-of-use filters, and valving. Since the definition of the system changes if any of these equipment components change, there must be a mechanism to identify when change has occurred. If this is a validated system, then the need to identify change can impact the need to revalidate.

Equipment numbers identify equipment. The format of an equipment identification number, however, can also be used to associate the equipment into a system. For example, if the equipment number is formatted as 00-AX-0000, where the first two digits are a system identification number and the last four digits are an equipment component identification number, then the association is made. Note: In this example the letters in the identification number are used to distinguish validated systems from unvalidated systems and systems that are maintained in-house from those on service contracts.

Once equipment systems are identified, their configuration should be documented. At a minimum this means that a specification sheet should be generated, containing a list of the equipment components, manufacturer, model number, capacity, and serial number. This listing should contain enough information about the equipment components to judge change when it occurs. For a validated system this listing should occur in the IQ document. If a system is not validated, similar configuration control may be appropriate.

These files can also be used to file equipment system requirements (i.e., what the systems are designed to do). Similarly, equipment specifications that describe how the equipment system fulfills the requirements would be appropriate for some systems. This document should describe what manual operations the automated system performs or replaces, what is monitored, what is controlled, and what type of data is collected. Describe the interrelationships of the data, data sequencing and processing, flowcharts, diagrams, and security.

In summary, the decision to make a list and/or create files for software and hardware components is a corporate decision. If there are only three computerized systems in the facility and sufficient control without identity numbers or files can be achieved, this is acceptable. The important point, however, is that the appropriate and sufficient control of these items IS demonstrated.

References

Agalloco, J. 1990. Computer System Validation Part III: Change Control. *BioPharm,* May:38–50.

Boogaard, P., and D. Epple. 1993. GLP Validation of Computer Systems: Vendor and End-User Responsibilities. *Pharmaceutical Engineering,* March/April:56–60.

Chamberlain, R. 1991. *Computer System Validation for the Pharmaceutical and Medical Device Industries.* Libertyville, IL: Alaren Press.

Christoff, S., and F. M. Sakers. 1993. Computer System Validation—Staying Current: Vendor-User Relationships. *BioPharm,* September:48–52.

Clark, A. S. 1988. Computer System Validation: An Investigator's View. *Pharmaceutical Technology,* January:60–65.

Costa, D. W., and J. W. Via. 1991. Configurable Software Validation for Batch Processes. *BioPharm,* May:40–45.

DeSain, C. V. 1991. Documentation Basics That Support Good Manufacturing Practices: Part Numbers. *BioPharm,* June:28–35.

DeSain, C. V. 1993. *Documentation Basics That Support Good Manufacturing Practices.* Cleveland: Advanstar Communications.

Donawa, M. E. 1992. Computer Software Validation and the US FDA (Part I). *Medical Device Technology,* November:12–20.

Donawa, M. E. 1992. Computer Software Validation and the US FDA (Part II). *Medical Device Technology,* December:10–13.

Erickson, J. R. 1993. Selecting Software for GMP Applications. *Medical Device and Diagnostic Industry,* January:122–128.

Goren, L. J. 1988. Computer System Validation Part I: Testing and Verification of Applications Software. *BioPharm,* November/December:28–35.

Goren, L. J. 1989. Computer System Validation Part II: Evaluating Vendor Software. *BioPharm,* February:38–43.

Guerra, J. 1988. Audits of Computer Systems in Analytical Laboratories. *Pharmaceutical Technology,* September:142–152.

Kuzel, N. R. 1987. Quality Assurance Auditing of Computer Systems. *Pharmaceutical Technology,* February:34–42.

Martensson, K. 1993. Prevalidation of Computer Systems Regulating Medical Device Manufacturing Processes. *Medical Device Technology,* April:22–25.

Schoenauer, C. M., and R. J. Wherry. 1993. Computer System Validation—Staying Current: Security in Computerized Systems. *Pharmaceutical Technology,* May:48–58.

Stotz, R. W., and K. G. Chapman. 1992. Validation of Automated Systems—System Definition. *Journal of Parenteral Science and Technology,* Vol. 43, No. 5:156–160.

Chapter 6

Process Validation

A process is the controlled interaction of components, equipment, environment, software, and personnel to produce a product or achieve an acceptable outcome. Process validation requires that the quality of the interacting components and the processing event be defined and controlled; an acceptable outcome of the process event should be described in product or process specifications **before** validation begins. The validation protocol simply describes a plan that demonstrates consistency in processing and confirms that all component, processing, and product specifications are appropriate and attainable under ideal and challenged conditions.

Cleaning, for example, is a process. The cleaning process is the interaction of chemicals, water, cleaning tools, objects to be cleaned, and people performing an established procedure to achieve clean areas, equipment, or products. To define and control the quality of the cleaning process, first identify the raw materials that are used (i.e., chemicals, water, buckets, sponges, and mops); define how people are trained in cleaning techniques; define the cleaning techniques that are appropriate for specific areas, equipment, or product; define what is considered an acceptable outcome; and define how it is measured or observed.

The validation of a defined and controlled cleaning process, as described above, becomes a simple demonstration of the interaction of materials, people, and equipment in a controlled manner to achieve a measurable or observable result. Cleaning validation would also include a demonstration of process reproducibility and ruggedness.

Process validation *must be performed* when

- The acceptability of processing cannot be fully measured or observed in the final product (e.g., sterilization).

Process validation *should be considered* when

- Processing directly affects product safety (e.g., sterility);

- Processing is significant, unique, or complex;

- The reliability of processing is unknown or suspect; and/or

- Routine monitoring or testing commitments could be minimized with a thorough demonstration of the validity of indicator testing.

Process validation should be performed when the process is fully developed and/or when the product of the process is manufactured for human use. Process validation, as with other validation events, is NOT an experiment or a process development project; process validation is an event that confirms that the established process can be performed reliably and consistently to produce a product of acceptable quality characteristics.

There are many processes that should be considered for qualification or validation in a medical product manufacturing facility. They can be logically divided into three general types: support, manufacturing, and product processes.

Support Processes

Support processes are processes that prepare materials, equipment, or environmental areas for the work of manufacturing. Support processes do not generally interact directly with final product. Support processes common to device manufacturing include room cleaning and disinfection, equipment sanitization, steam-in-place and clean-in-place operations, inventory control, and material preparation and processing events.

Standard Manufacturing Processes

Manufacturing processes are standard events used to process many products. They are often equipment dependent; they can include assembly, formulation, mixing, curing, coating, drilling, crimping, soldering, product or component cleaning, sterilization, sealing, packaging, labeling, and inspection.

These manufacturing processes can be qualified (IQ and OQ) for use with a range of products, and then individual products can be qualified or validated with these manufacturing processes, when appropriate. A product qualification event, for example, would be a single demonstration that the product performs as expected with the qualified manufacturing process. A product validation event, for example, would demonstrate reproducibility of the manufacturing process under ideal and challenged conditions with the qualified manufacturing process.

Product Processes

A product processing event is a manufacturing process that is product specific. Each configuration of standard manufacturing process events can be unique for each product. In one product, for example, an assembly event may be followed by a curing step and another assembly step before final packaging and sterilization. In another product there may be a cleaning step after the final assembly event. Whatever the configuration of manufacturing processes, it is a process that is unique to each product. Product validation, as a result, is a terminal event, performed after the qualification or validation of the subprocessing events.

Product validation must demonstrate the consistency and reliability of the product manufacturing event from beginning to end with multiple units or lots of product (at least three are expected). The acceptance criteria for this validation event must ensure that all processing parameters meet specifications and that the final product meets specifications.

Product Validation vs. Design Verification

The validation of the product manufacturing event should be performed when the product design is completed. Validation is not a tool of the development engineer; it is a tool of the manufacturing engineer. This is a point of great confusion in the industry.

Validation is a terminal event to the development process. In some corporations it is performed by the development group; in other organizations it is performed by the manufacturing group. Although the delegation of responsibility is not as important as the proper performance of the work, there are inherent difficulties in performing validation in the development group or department.

Development engineers or scientists are trained to develop and improve processes and products. They are, as a result, always changing things to achieve that end. Validation, however, is not a development process; it is not an experiment. It is a planned evaluation of an established process that confirms that the process can be performed as directed and produce acceptable product.

During validation one **cannot change** the components, raw materials, processing events, process acceptance criteria, final product design or configuration, or final product acceptance criteria. Also, during validation the work must be performed in the location and with the equipment that will be used for commercial manufacturing. As a result, these two requirements make it very difficult to perform validation events in the development laboratory.

Much of the confusion comes from an inappropriate use of terminology. The design development group must verify the safety and performance of the product as it develops. This testing, inspection, and review is appropriately called design verification rather than design validation.

Typically, a product and its manufacturing process are developed by design development. After design verification has been completed, the product is released for clinical trials and/or commercial production. This release may involve a new site of manufacture, new manufacturing equipment, a larger scale of manufacturing, and new personnel. Whatever the differences between design-development manufacturing and commercial-scale manufacturing, change usually occurs. It must be demonstrated that this change does not adversely affect the quality of the product or the quality of the manufacturing process. Validation can provide this assurance.

Categorization of Processes

Validation is not appropriate for all processing events. To facilitate the validation of processing events, therefore, processes should be categorized according to their potential affect on the safety and performance of the product. Three categories—I, II, III—are usually sufficient.

Category III Processes require validation. The failure or inconsistent performance of these processes could adversely affect the safety or effectiveness of the product. These processes must include product sterilization, product depyrogenation, and aseptic processing events of product that will not be terminally sterilized; the effectiveness of these processing events cannot be adequately tested in the final product. Consider Category III for any processing event that affects the safety of the product to the patient, consumer, or user; safety issues include electrical, radiation, mechanical, chemical, and biological. Consider Category III for processing events that directly affect the performance of the product when that performance is life supporting or the information provided by the product (e.g. a diagnostic product) is the sole source of information for a critical treatment decision. Finally, consider Category III for processing events whose outcome could directly and significantly affect the uniformity or reliability of the product.

Category II Processes require qualification. This means that the components interacting in the process must be identified and controlled and that the process itself must be established in a controlled document such as an SOP or device manufacturing record (DMR). Qualification of a process requires a demonstration that the process can be performed effectively, but there is not a demonstration of process consistency under ideal and challenged conditions. An automated packaging process for a nonsterile product, for example, may require qualification but not validation.

The reliability of Category I Processes can be assured with controlled documentation, training of personnel, and simple equipment calibration and preventive maintenance procedures. If they are automated processes, however, they may be appropriate for Category II.

Process Validation Protocol: Format and Content

The format and content of a process validation protocol should be determined by the manufacturer. Consider the following format and content suggestions:

Purpose

Describe the purpose of the process validation or qualification event (i.e., why is this evaluation necessary?). Is it a retrospective, concurrent, or prospective validation or some combination of these?

Scope

Describe which processing events this protocol addresses. If identical processing events occur in both the production and the development departments, or if identical processing events occur in more than one location, describe how this protocol applies to each.

Responsibility

Who is responsible for writing the protocol, performing the work, and reviewing/approving the data package?

Process History

If the process was developed in-house, make reference to development reports and/or turnover packages. Is the process new? Is this an existing process that has had a change of status recently, requiring validation? Whatever the history of the process, briefly describe it.

Process Description/Flow

Describe how the product moves through the process and the facility. If appropriate, provide a flow diagram indicating the location of each step of the process; if appropriate, provide batching or pooling considerations and any time sequence requirements.

Processing Variables/Controls

List the processing variables, the methods used to measure these variables, and the limits of acceptability. Each variable should have a minimum and maximum acceptable value. Ensure that the significant numbers in the units of measure for acceptance criteria can be supported by the accuracy and precision of the method.

The Processing Record

Before any process can be validated, the processing procedure must be defined and documented. The procedure document must describe the processing event in a step-by-step manner, providing for sampling and testing points. It must identify raw materials, equipment, and utility and environmental requirements. A DMR should indicate processing parameters, methods to assess them, acceptance criteria, and yield or accountability when appropriate.

Worst Case Challenge and Rationale

Describe how the processing event will be challenged. This challenge should be representative of the extremes of acceptable conditions, demonstrating that the process continues to perform reliably. It is not necessary to perform an endless number of challenge events; rather it is instructive to determine what extremes are appropriate and what conditions best challenge the reliability of the processing event.

Validation

Preliminary Operations

Describe what calibration, qualification, or validation events need to be completed before this process validation begins. Describe any material processing events that must be completed before the validation begins. Describe any technician training that must be completed.

Process Qualification

Describe what will be done (i.e., the process that will be qualified) or reference the SOP or DMR document number and revision number that will be used. Declare the number of times the event will be performed (e.g., three consecutive events). Describe what is considered an acceptable outcome for both processing parameters and product.

Product Qualification

Describe how much product will be manufactured, how many manufacturing events will be performed to demonstrate consistency and reliability, and what is considered an acceptable outcome for both processing parameters and product.

Validation Acceptance Criteria

Describe the overall acceptance criteria for the validation event. This should include a commitment to account for data and review data for accuracy and completeness. A validation is approved only when both the processing parameters and the product meet specifications and when the documentation to support the event is complete and acceptable.

Routine Monitoring Commitments

Describe the monitoring and control requirements that will ensure, routinely, that the process continues to perform within the limits of validation.

Product Reliability Test Commitments

If product from the validation event is placed into reliability or stability test programs, reference these commitments.

Documentation Requirements

Describe how the data derived from the performance of this protocol will be recorded, reviewed, approved, and filed.

Process Change Control

Once a process is established and documented in writing, any change to that process must be controlled. The significance of the process change and its potential impact on the safety, performance, uniformity, and reliability of final product must be considered before the change is implemented. If the process has been qualified or validated, then the impact of the change may include the need for revalidation. This will be discussed in chapters 11 and 12.

References

Agalloco, J. 1992. Points to Consider in the Validation of Equipment Cleaning Procedures. *Journal of Parenteral Science and Technology,* September/October:163–168.

DeSain, C. V. 1993. *Drug, Device and Diagnostic Manufacturing: The Ultimate Resource Handbook.* 2nd ed. Buffalo Grove, IL: Interpharm Press.

How Clean is Clean? Validation of Cleaning Procedures in Manufacturing Equipment. Bern: European Organization for Quality.

Prince, R. 1993. EPA and FDA Efficacy-Testing Requirements for Chemical Germicides and Reprocessed Devices. *Medical Device and Diagnostic Industry,* May:152–160.

Zeller, A. O. 1993. Cleaning Validation and Residue Limits: A Contribution to Current Discussions. *Pharmaceutical Technology,* October:70–80.

Chapter 7

Documentation: The Tools of Validation

The documentation of validation is fundamental. The documents must be clearly written and organized in a manner that makes validation work flow logically and quickly. Validation is a rigorous task; the efficiency of the validation process, as a result, significantly impacts the cost of manufacturing.

Protocols, plans, procedures, specifications, device manufacturing records, forms, reports, and logbooks are the tools of validation. The validation plan or protocol must be written before the work begins. These commitment documents must be supported by documents that direct the work (i.e., procedures, specifications, device manufacturing records, or production batch records). Similarly, these directive documents must be supported by data collection documents that facilitate the collection of data and assure its accuracy and completeness. The commitment documents, the directive documents, and the data collection documents must be controlled, meaning that their issue and change is a reviewed and approved process.

The Validation Master Plan

When the validation commitment is large or complex, one should organize the commitments to validation in a Validation Master

Plan. This document describes the overall corporate commitment to validation and further defines commitments to equipment, method, software, and process validation. An example Validation Master Plan is provided in the appendix to this chapter.

Validation Protocols

Validation protocols are controlled documents that describe how to perform a validation event. They can reference standard operating procedures, specifications, and device manufacturing records as appropriate. They must contain or reference the acceptance criteria for the events they direct. An example follows at the end of this chapter; note, however, that this protocol would require forms to record the data and observations that it directs.

Validation Reports

Validation reports are narrative summaries of a specific validation event. They should reference the validation protocol document identification number and its revision level, as well as any identification numbers specific for the equipment, utility system, process, or software evaluated. These reports summarize data and declare the disposition of the item validated.

Validation Notebooks/Validation Files

The validation protocol, the raw data, and the validation report should be assembled in a notebook or file to facilitate review and approval. Each validation event should generate a notebook or file. These are controlled documents that should be stored in a secure area. They must be readily available for review, however, by regulatory authorities, potential clients, and so on. Every time a validation is repeated, a new file or notebook is generated, even if the same revision level of the same protocols is used or followed. In the case of revalidation events, however, the validation report should indicate the reason and the rationale for the event.

Validation Certificates

When a validation event is finished, when the report has been written, and when the validation data has been reviewed by management, a certificate should be issued declaring the acceptability or unacceptability of the validation and its expiration date, if appropriate. Validations can fail, and this must be an option on the validation certificate.

The validation certificate should indicate what documents have been reviewed, the results of testing, and any deviations or out-of-specification results that were investigated during the course of validation. These certificates must declare a disposition of the validation event and must be signed by responsible individuals. The certificate should appear in the validation notebook. When possible, a validation sticker should appear on or near the equipment that has been validated, indicating the date of validation and the date of expiration.

Chapter Appendix:
The Validation Master Plan—An Example

1.0 Purpose

This document describes the Our Laboratories, Inc. (OLI), commitment to validation and provides an overview of how that commitment will be implemented.

2.0 Scope

This document presents general guidelines for the development of a validation plan for equipment, utility systems, analytical methods, software, and critical processing events used to produce products for human use at the OLI manufacturing facility in Tofte, MN.

3.0 Responsibility

The validation plan will be designed, coordinated, and implemented by the Validation Department as defined in this document.

4.0 Protocol

Validation is an exercise that results in documented evidence, with a high degree of assurance, that a specific utility system, equipment, method, or process will consistently produce "product" meeting predetermined specifications and quality characteristics. The product may be water from a WFI system, steam from a steam generator, an assay result, or final product for human use.

Validation activities must be planned, and validation protocols must be designed, reviewed, and approved in order to assure that the evidence collected does, in fact, demonstrate consistent, reliable performance/operation.

4.1 The Validation Committee

Since validation requires technical knowledge from many different disciplines and ultimately has an impact on every major function in a manufacturing facility, all departments should be involved in validation planning and decision making. The OLI Validation Department plans, coordinates, and implements validation activities.

The department is responsible for

- Determining what will require validation
- Determining the level of evaluation (as discussed below)
- Writing the validation plan
- Designing validation protocols
- Writing, reviewing, and approving validation protocols
- Scheduling and coordinating the work of validation
- Resolving problems encountered during validation
- Compiling/reviewing/approving data generated from validation events
- Writing validation report summaries
- Determining when revalidation is appropriate

4.2 The Validation Assessment/Plan

There are several reasons why validation may be required:

- New facilities, new equipment, or new product lines
- Modification/change in equipment, methods, processing, or products
- Scale-up of a process
- Scheduled revalidation

The Validation Department must write a plan for each major validation event. The plan must list the utilities, equipment, methods, processes, or products that will be validated, why validation is required, the rationale for the rigor of validation, scheduling requirements, and how the validation will be carried out (protocol or SOP references). In addition, the plan must consider and describe any impact that validation may have on existing or subsequent lots of product.

This plan can be in memo form, but the original plan must be signed by QA, Production, and Validation. This plan will be identified by the date of initial issue. Amendments to the plan will always reference the original date.

4.3 Types of Validation

Validation activities logically fall into four categories or types of work: utility or equipment validation, analytical method validation, software validation, and process/product validation. The category distinctions are based primarily on the fundamental differences in the format and content of the validation protocols. The guidelines for format, content, review, approval, and control of specific validation protocols are presented in

- MP02: Master Utility/Equipment Validation Plan

- MP03: Master Method Validation Plan

- MP04: Master Process Validation Plan

- MP05: Master Software Validation Plan

4.4 Levels of Validation/Qualification

Validation at OLI means a full evaluation of a method, process, software, product, or equipment system. According to the traditional definitions of validation for equipment and utility systems, for example, this includes an installation qualification (IQ), an operational qualification (OQ) and a performance qualification (PQ).

Not all equipment, methods, processes, and utility systems, however, may require a full validation to demonstrate consistent and reliable performance/operation. A house steam system, for example, may require only an IQ and OQ evaluation. Similarly, a well-recognized protein assay may require only the use of proper controls and standards. Any evaluation meant to provide documented evidence that equipment, methods, or processes will consistently perform/operate and that **does not** require a full validation is called a **qualification.**

Determining what requires qualification and what requires validation is the responsibility of the Validation Department and should be declared in the Master Validation Plan. These decisions should be based on the affect that the "product" of the equipment, method, or process will have on the safety, purity, efficacy, or stability of the final product and on the uniqueness of the equipment, method, or process.

Categorization guidelines are discussed in the validation plans (MP02, MP03, MP04, MP05).

4.5 The Validation Protocol

A validation protocol is a written plan that describes how to conduct validation activities and how to measure the success of the process, method, or equipment performance. It identifies raw materials, key processing variables, intermediates, and final product acceptance criteria. Each validation event must be conducted according to this written plan.

The validation protocol is a controlled document and is created, issued, and controlled according to the guidelines in the validation plans (MP02, MP03, MP04, MP05).

4.6 Validation Protocol Amendments

While performing the tasks directed in a validation protocol, especially for a new system, a new piece of equipment, or a new method or process, it is not uncommon to learn things during the event that require changes in the protocol. In this case it is not appropriate to change the protocol through formal change control procedures and reissue it, as this would result in a protocol signed and approved after the completion of validation tasks.

It is appropriate, however, to issue an amendment to the protocol that describes the changes and the rationale for change. These amendments, which can be in memo format, must be approved by the Validation Department and QA.

4.7 Scheduling Validation Events

The validation of an entire facility is a very complex task, and the order of validation has a significant impact on the effectiveness of this evaluation process. Equipment must be validated before processes that use it are validated. For example, steam systems must be validated before any equipment that utilizes steam is validated. Water systems must be validated before steam systems.

The Validation Department is responsible for scheduling validation events, whether for a new facility, a new product line, or an individual revalidation event.

4.8 Deviations/Investigations That Occur During Validation

Any deviations that occur during the performance of a validation event must be reviewed by the Validation Department. If an investigation is initiated, it must have the approval of the committee, and they must review and accept the results of this investigation. All investigations must be documented.

4.9 Validation Data Review/Approval Requirements

When a validation event is completed, the data is compiled and reviewed for accuracy by Quality Assurance. The Validation Department reviews the data and determines whether or not the results are acceptable. A summary report is written; copies are provided to the VP of Operations for the corporation and any other appropriate executives.

If the validation is acceptable, a validation certificate is issued, indicating that the item is validated, the protocol number and revision level, the date that validation is completed, and the date that revalidation is scheduled. Validation certificates must be signed by QA, Maintenance, Production, and Validation. These signatures indicate that each member finds the results of the validation acceptable. If appropriate, validation certificates are posted on equipment or near processing lines.

4.10 Revalidation Guidelines

Validation events must be repeated periodically to ensure that the systems remain unchanged. These revalidation events can be triggered by a change in the equipment, utility, method, or process, or by the passage of time without change.

As a general rule, revalidation, as defined in individual protocols, will be scheduled every 12–18 months. At this time data collected from the routine use or processing of the equipment, method, or process will be reviewed and appropriate evaluation criteria will be determined by the Validation Department. When appropriate, validation protocols are revised to prepare for the next validation event.

4.11 Documentation Requirements

A validation notebook is compiled for each validation event, containing the relevant copy of the protocol, the summary report, and summary and/or raw data to support the tasks directed in the protocol.

References

DeSain, C. V. 1993. *Documentation Basics That Support Good Manufacturing Practices.* Cleveland: Advanstar Communications.

DeSain, C. V. 1992. Documentation Basics That Support Good Manufacturing Practices: Equipment and Utility System Validation Protocols. *BioPharm,* May:21–34.

DeSain, C. V. 1992. Documentation Basics That Support Good Manufacturing Practices: Master Method Validation Protocols. *BioPharm,* June:30–34.

DeSain, C. V. 1992. Documentation Basics That Support Good Manufacturing Practices: Process Validation Protocols. *BioPharm,* July–August:22–24.

Chapter 8

Validation of Device Manufacturing in a One-Product Facility

In this chapter we will examine the operation of a small device manufacturer and help determine the validation requirements associated with its product. Tofte Medical (TM) is a small company with fifteen employees. It was incorporated 3 years ago for the sole purpose of providing a new coated drainage catheter to the market.

Tofte Medical is located in an industrial complex. They rent 10,000 square feet of office space, which has been subdivided into a laboratory/test area and a production area that includes a clean room and packaging, shipping, receiving, and administrative areas. Currently, both design development and QC work together in the same laboratory area. The production area was recently remodeled and the clean room was upgraded from a laminar flow hood to a limited-access area. This upgrade was initiated to comply with the expectations of Good Manufacturing Practices and to accommodate the scale-up demands of commercial manufacturing.

The product is classified as Class II, according to the FDA; TM has recently filed an IDE application with the FDA. As a result, all product manufactured in the facility from this point forward is available for human use. In anticipation of this event, management has handed down a facility-wide mandate for GMP compliance.

You have been recently hired as Production Manager; in addition, TM has hired an experienced QA Manager. The Development Manager is one of the original founders of the company, and he has decided that the GMPs do not apply to him or his department. You try not to antagonize this man and instead focus on your mission (i.e., to set up the Production Department and validate the manufacturing process).

In order to determine appropriate and reasonable validation commitments, you ask to watch a manufacturing event in the Development Laboratory from beginning to end. You ask the new QA Manager for a copy of the procedures or records that describe the event, and you obtain a copy of the Manufacturing and Control Section of the IDE.

Processing Overview

What is the manufacturing process? What are the major steps in the manufacture of a coated drainage catheter? Who performs the work? What controls are currently in place to assure the success of each processing step? How is the success of each processing step measured or determined? Have there been any problems associated with processing? What processing changes are planned for the new facility?

In an attempt to answer these questions, you observe a catheter manufacturing event, review existing documentation, and talk with Development and QA. Then you compile the following information:

Plastic Tubing Extrusion

This is performed outside the corporation at Pulaski Plastics, according to specifications provided by TM; material is currently received and used without test or inspection. No problems have been associated with this component; the vendor will be able to support scale-up demands.

Tube Cutting

This is a manual process performed by a technician with a razor blade. Cut tubes are racked in holders marked with tolerances and there is, as a result, a 100 percent visual check of each tube. No problems have been associated with this processing step, and no changes are anticipated for scale-up.

Forming Tip Taper and Curve

Cut tubing is heated in a thermal former. The curve and the taper are formed using a preformed wire and a heated die—a manual operation that will remain manual with scale-up. A dedicated thermal former will be purchased for this processing event with scale-up. Problems associated with this processing event include incomplete forming, pits and voids in the heated section of tubing, and tip hole blockage.

Drilling of Holes

Each tube is placed in a jig and three holes are drilled manually. Each drilled subassembly is inspected by a technician for cleanliness and edge smoothness. There have been no significant problems associated with this processing event. This process will remain manual with scale-up.

Assembly, Adhesion, and Curing of Luer Adapters and Tubing

A luer fitting is attached to the tubing with an adhesive, and then the assemblies are cured in an oven at established time and temperature settings determined during product development. This entire process is manual. The current oven, however, is used for several curing operations and it is not uncommon to see more than one type of catheter in the oven at the same time. Currently, the oven door cannot be secured against unscheduled entry.

The adequacy of this curing step is assured with a pull test performed with a tensile tester on a 10 percent sampling of each cured lot.

A dedicated oven has been ordered for this processing step. The oven door can be secured during a timed cycle.

Cleaning of Assembly

A manual flush and rinse is performed with alcohol and water, delivered from a pressurized tube. The pressure of the water has not been previously known or controlled, but will be in the new facility. Water for injection is purchased for this event.

The QA Manager says that no SOP exists for the cleaning step and, therefore, no rinse time has been established. The engineers claim that cleaning is performed to remove extrusion agents, particulates, mold release compounds, and bioburden.

Tube Coating

The coating process occurs in dip tanks. The tank size and configuration will remain the same with scale-up. There will simply be more units processed in the tank. After three coating cycles the formulation tank is cleaned and the chemicals are changed.

A quick review of the SOP and device manufacturing record that accompanies this event suggests that not all of the critical parameters associated with the event are adequately controlled. Current testing includes a visual inspection of the coating for discoloration, flaking, and irregularities; coat thickness is measured destructively. There is no test method available to determine the uniformity of the coating layer.

Drying

The drying step is designed to allow the coating material to cure. The development engineers insist that there are no time or temperature limits for this process because the coating will cure eventually. (Nevertheless, you understand that the process must be controlled and have asked them to investigate a method to determine the extent of curing.)

Testing

During this testing event product is inspected for length, proper configuration, quantity and size of holes, curve and taper diameter, attachment of luer, cleanliness, and coating integrity, according to a sampling plan. Bioburden is performed according to SOP 222 by an outside testing laboratory.

Heat Sealing and Labeling

The heat sealing process will be upgraded with the new facility to a tray with a Tyvek® cover. These units can be sealed, six units at a time in the new heat sealing unit. There are settings for time, temperature, and pressure.

Sterilization

Ethylene oxide sterilization is performed at an outside contractor. The sterilization contractor claims to already have validated cycles for the new configuration of the product, although TM's product has not been tested directly. There have been no known problems with this contractor, and they seem willing and able to support scale-up to commercial production lots; however, TM has not officially audited this contractor.

Testing

All final product testing is performed in-house, except for sterility testing. The latter is performed by the same contractor that performs the sterilization event.

Labeling

Labels, which are currently applied manually, will be changed to preprinted Tyvek® lids for the tray. The Tyvek® will be hot stamped with the lot number before application.

Documentation Review

QA has assumed the responsibility for upgrading the documentation for the processing **before** validation begins. They expect, however, that you, as Production Manager, can easily provide an accurate description of the manufacturing process.

You look at the documents that exist currently. Every production event at TM is directed with a standard operating procedure—actually several SOPs—and the results of the work are recorded on a device history form. While observing the processing events, however, you noticed that the records no longer accurately describe the work. This seems to be because the SOPs are not usually open on the bench where the technician works, and if they are, they are not consulted.

You decide, as a result, to incorporate all product-specific instructions from the procedures into the device manufacturing record. For example, the operation of the heat sealing unit will remain in a SOP document, but the settings appropriate for this product will appear in the device manufacturing record. This will minimize the redundancy of information and ensure that the information the technician needs to perform the work accurately is immediately available.

Training Review

Clearly, technicians need to be trained to follow written instructions. They have learned to ignore them at TM, mostly because they knew that the instructions were wrong. When the new documents are drafted, a major GMP training program will be initiated by Quality Assurance. In addition, you will begin task-specific training for production workers.

Facility Construction and Equipment Installation

The facility upgrade has resulted in significant changes to the basic utility systems (i.e., the compressed air system has been replaced and a limited-access clean room area has been installed). This work was completed before you started at TM, and the installation documentation that you expect to find is not on file in the facility.

A development engineer has recently been assigned to production, part-time, and you decide to give this engineer the authority and responsibility to design and implement preventive maintenance programs and calibration programs for all equipment (i.e., utility systems, production equipment, and test equipment). In addition, this engineer will obtain "as-built" blueprints of the HVAC system and the compressed air systems from the contractors. All installation documentation (i.e. calibration events, cleaning events, and performance tests) will be filed at TM. User manuals and repair manuals will also be on file.

Validation Planning

Although you have been given the authority and responsibility to validate the manufacturing process, that responsibility was given with the warning that you should "only do what you have to do."

Given your timeline, you agree with that philosophy, but you also know that you will be held accountable for specific 483 citations resulting from an FDA inspection.

So you decide to make your validation decisions based on the collective knowledge of the current reliability of TM processing events, the projected impact of increased production levels, the critical nature of the processing, and the definition of "special processes" in the new GMPs.

You call a meeting of the managers and after several hours of discussion, you agree, generally to validate and qualify individual processing events, test methods and equipment, when appropriate, and then to perform a product validation event to confirm the reproducibility of the entire production process and the consistency of final product. The rigor of these evaluations will be categorized as described in previous chapters (i.e., Category I, II, and III.)

Process Validation Commitments

A list of processing events that will require a complete validation (Category III) is proposed. There is no argument about the need to validate the catheter manufacturing process. In addition, there is no argument about the validation of significant subprocesses that can directly affect the safety of the device (i.e., sterilization of final product, the heat sealing process, or the sterility test procedure). There is, however, heated discussion about the proposal to validate the tube coating process and the subassembly cleaning process.

Tube Coating

Why should TM validate the tube coating process? Does anyone else do this? Is this a special process? Every lot of catheters is inspected routinely; what good is validation? Can the final product be evaluated adequately for the effectiveness of this coating process?

You attempt to lead this discussion by asking questions. The first question concerns safety issues associated with the coating process:

What could go wrong? Could a poorly coated tube hurt a patient?

Everyone seems to agree that it is possible. If portions of the coating separated from the tubing, it could flake off into the patient. The group understands that because safety issues are at stake, validation must be considered. But is this a special process? Do current testing requirements sufficiently assess the acceptability of the tube coat?

What are the characteristics of a good coat?

- Uniformity of coating consistency over catheter length

- Uniformity of coating thickness over catheter length

- A predetermined stiffness or flexibility over catheter length

- Adherence of the coating to the plastic tubing, under worst case and throughout shelf life

How do we currently test for these characteristics?

- Uniformity is assessed by visual examination.

- Stiffness and flexibility is tested.

- There is no test for coating adherence to the tubing.

Does visual examination detect poorly coated catheters? Does the stiffness/flexibility testing detect poorly coated catheters? Is there a simple way to test for adherence? Could a catheter that passes stiffness/flexibility tests and visual inspection deteriorate during sterilization or over its shelf life to injure a patient? Is this likely to happen?

What aspects of the processing itself could affect the adherence or uniformity of the coat?

The positive outcome of this discussion was the realization that there needs to be more control of the coating process. It was agreed that the tank solution would be changed based on time and on usage. A maximum of three uses would be allowed before new solution was formulated. An expiration date of one week would be assigned to the coating solution once it was formulated in the tank. In addition, a SOP was written describing how to clean the tank between uses.

Given that formulated coating solution could layer in the tank with time, the need to mix the tank before the coating event begins was then discussed. A mixer will be installed before validation begins.

Finally, the group decided that validation would be useful if it could demonstrate the adequacy of the minimal testing routine (i.e., visual inspection and flexibility/stiffness tests to assure coat uniformity and adherence). A protocol was proposed. One batch of catheters, meaning one dip-tank run, would be processed in newly formulated coating solution; one batch would be processed in used coating solution; one batch would be processed in one-week-old coating solution that had been used twice previously.

In addition to routine release tests, an increased sampling of product would be tested for uniformity at three intervals over its length and an adherence stress test would be developed to test the product initially and over its shelf life. Acceptance criteria for all testing would appear in the protocol.

Subassembly Cleaning Process

Should cleaning be validated? What is the purpose of cleaning? How do we know if cleaning is effective?

This discussion results in the realization that no one has ever really looked at or thought about cleaning. No one knows how dirty the catheters are before they are cleaned, and no one knows how much "less dirty" they are, if at all, after they are cleaned. It just seemed like a good thing to do; it has always been a part of the processing. In fact there is no standard for "how clean is clean enough."

It is decided that TM must first determine what contaminants and impurities are on the subassembly, then what level of these contaminants or impurities is acceptable. Next TM must determine if the current cleaning procedure is appropriate and adequate. If final product testing does not adequately assess cleaning effectiveness, TM will consider validation.

The outcome of this development work ultimately resulted in the decision not to validate cleaning. The cleaning process, by that time, had been well developed, additional process controls were instituted to ensure consistency in the cleaning procedures, and a test was introduced for the final product to determine its cleanliness.

This discussion, in general, made the group realize that although the product had been developed through the development process at TM, the manufacturing **process** had not been fully developed. Validation decisions are difficult when manufacturing processes are not appropriately controlled and when the effectiveness of a manufacturing process is not adequately measured.

Process Qualification Commitments

The group quickly agreed on the following list of processes and equipment requiring an installation and operational qualification (Category II):

Equipment

Compressed air system
Drying and curing oven
Clean room

Processes

UV light curing
Labeling
Extrusion (at contractor)

An example protocol for the qualification of the hot air oven is provided in the appendix to this chapter.

Calibration and Preventive Maintenance Commitments

The group reviewed the manufacturing process and testing commitments for the catheter and made the following list of items that must be calibrated before the product validation event:

Tensile tester
Thermal former
Drill
Calipers
Hot stamper

Product Validation Commitments

Product validation is planned when the

- Process control commitments, discussed above, are complete;
- Qualification and calibration events, discussed above, are complete;

- Manufacturing record and SOP documents are approved; and

- GMP training of employees is completed.

Product validation requires that the product of the validation event be made from beginning to end as it is routinely manufactured for commercial use. This means that product must be manufactured in the same facility, with the same equipment, with the same technicians, with the same raw materials, and at the same scale or lot size as will be used routinely. If it is not, then the need to revalidate when processing is moved to full-scale, commercial production must be considered.

A minimum of three runs or lots of product, of the same batch size, are manufactured to demonstrate consistency. *Consistency* means that the processing parameters must regularly meet predetermined specifications and that the product meets predetermined specifications.

There has been disagreement at TM about the need to control catheter batch size. One batch size was chosen, however, because it represents the largest number of catheters that can be processed identically through the coating process and yet is the minimum number of catheters that will be manufactured in the new facility during a single production event.

The product validation protocol is designed to challenge the following three aspects of routine processing:

1. There is sometimes a delay of up to 24 hours between tube coating and tube drying. As a result, the validation event will dry one run of product immediately after coating and one run of product will be held for 24 hours at room temperature before it is dried in the oven.

2. Three different lots of plastic tubing will be used to manufacture the three different lots of catheters for this validation event. Two different lots of adhesive will be used. There are two different approved vendors for the Tyvek® pouches; both will be used during validation.

3. All employees qualified to work on this processing line will participate in this validation event.

Summary

From the example provided in this chapter, it should be evident that it is difficult, if not impossible, to validate an incompletely developed product. Similarly, it is difficult, if not impossible, to validate an incompletely developed manufacturing process. When product and process development are complete, however, validation is a simple exercise that confirms the ability of the manufacturing process to consistently produce product of established quality characteristics. Validation is the beginning of process control programs that will routinely assure process and product consistency.

Another lesson from the example provided in this chapter is that unless final product can be adequately tested for the effectiveness of subprocessing events, one should consider qualification or validation of the subprocesses before one performs a product validation. If the subprocessing event contributes to or provides product safety characteristics, then validation is highly recommended. If the subprocessing event contributes to or provides product performance characteristics that cannot be adequately assessed by final product testing, then subprocess validation is recommended.

Chapter Appendix:
Hot Air Oven Qualification Protocol—
An Example

1.0 Purpose

This protocol describes how to qualify a hot air oven for curing and drying steps in the manufacture of drainage catheters.

2.0 Scope

This protocol applies to the Gruenberg hot air oven, Model 345T, in the TM facility used in the GMP production of drainage catheters for human use.

3.0 Responsibility

The oven qualification is performed by production. The qualification results are reported, reviewed, and approved by the validation committee.

4.0 Protocol

During drainage catheter production the hot air oven is used for curing epoxied joints and for drying and curing coated drainage catheters. This qualification is designed, therefore, to cover the range of operation common to these processing events.

   This oven is newly installed.

4.1 Installation Qualification

Establish and document that the oven is properly installed. Complete an installation qualification document as directed in SOP 333.

4.2 Operational Qualification

- **Calibration:** Calibrate thermocouples according to SOP 222. Calibrate chart recorder according to SOP 311. Calibrate timer according to SOP 421.

- **Alarm settings:** Set the oven temperature above the high temperature alarm setting of 250°C. Verify that the alarm sounds when the temperature exceeds 250°C.

- **Safety features:** Verify that the oven door locks when the cycle is in progress.

- **Electromechanical functions:** Program the oven for a time and temperature cycle setting. Run the oven. Verify that the chart recorder functions properly and that the cycle recorded matches the cycle set.

- **Heat distribution (empty chamber):** Perform the heat distribution assessment within 30 days of the calibration of thermocouples.

- **Placement of thermocouples:** Place TCs in an X pattern throughout the chamber.

- **Cycle settings:** There are two cycle settings: one representing a drying cycle and one representing the curing cycle.

  — Cycle A = 250°C, 4 hours

  — Cycle B = 125°C, 6 hours

- **Cycle performance:** Run three cycles at setting A and three cycles at setting B. Collect TC data at 15-minute intervals.

- **Data collection:** Collect the chart recorder from each cycle. Collect thermocouple data from each cycle at 15-minute intervals.

- **Acceptance criteria for heat distribution cycle:**

  — The chart recorder must indicate that the oven during Cycle A was at 235–265°C for $3^3/_4$ hours to $4^1/_2$ hours.

  — The chart recorder must indicate that the oven during Cycle B was at 115–140°C for $5^3/_4$ hours to $6^1/_2$ hours.

  All thermocouples must read within 10°C of one another at any given time point. The thermocouple in the cold spot must meet the criteria for the chart recorders presented above.

- **Calibration of thermocouples:** Upon completion of the study, calibrate the thermocouples according to SOP 222.

5.0 Acceptance Criteria for Qualification

The calibration of thermocouples, timers and chart recorders meets specifications established in the equipment files for these items. The alarms function properly. The safety features of the unit operate properly. All heat distribution studies meet acceptance criteria.

References

Agalloco, J. 1993. The Validation Life Cycle. *Journal of Parenteral Science and Technology,* May–June:142–147.

ANSI/AAMI Guideline for Industrial EtO Sterilization of Medical Devices: Process Design, Validation, Routine Sterilization and Contract Sterilization. ST27-1988.

Application of the Medical Device GMPs to Computerized Devices and Manufacturing Processes: Medical Device GMP Guidance for FDA Investigators, first draft. 11/90. Rockville, MD: CDRH.

Chapman, K. G. 1991. A History of Validation in the United States: Part I. *Pharmaceutical Technology,* October:82–96.

Compliance Program 7382.830A, Sterilization of Medical Devices. 9/91. Rockville, MD: FDA.

DeSain, C. V. 1993. *Documentation Basics That Support Good Manufacturing Practices.* Cleveland: Advanstar Communications.

DeSain, C. V. 1993. *Drug, Device and Diagnostic Manufacturing: The Ultimate Resource Handbook.* 2nd ed. Buffalo Grove, IL: Interpharm Press.

DeSain, C. V., and C. L. Vercimak. 1994. *Implementing International GMPs for Drug, Device, and Diagnostic Manufacturers: A Practical Guide.* Buffalo Grove, IL: Interpharm Press.

DeVecchi, F. 1986. Validation of Air Systems Used in Parenteral Drug Manufacturing Facilities. In *Validation of Aseptic Pharmaceutical Processes,* F. J. Carleton and J. P. Agalloco, eds., 125–162. New York: Marcel Dekker.

FDA Medical Device Regulation from Premarket Review to Recall. 1991. Rockville, MD: DHHS, Office of Inspector General.

Garfinkle, B. D. 1986. Validation of Utilities. In *Validation of Aseptic Pharmaceutical Processes,* F. J. Carleton and J. P. Agalloco, eds., 185–205. New York: Marcel Dekker.

Guideline for the Manufacturing of IVD Products. 1/94. Rockville, MD: FDA/CDRH.

Guidelines on the General Principles of Process Validation. 1987. Rockville, MD: FDA.

Implementing the Good Manufacturing Practices Regulation. *U.S. General Accounting Office Testimony,* March 25, 1992, GAO/T-PEMD-92-6.

Medical Device GMP Guidance for FDA Investigators. DHHS Publication FDA 84-4191, April, 1987. Rockville, MD: CDRH.

Medical Device GMP Manual. 1991. 5th ed. Rockville, MD: Division of Small Manufacturer's Assistance, FDA/CDRH, 91-4179.

Preproduction Quality Assurance Planning: Recommendations for Medical Device Manufacturers. HHS Publication FDA 90-4236, 9/89. Rockville, MD: CDRH.

Suggested Changes to Medical Device Regulations: Information Document. 11/90. Rockville, MD: CDRH.

Technical Report: Software Development Activities: Reference Materials and Training Aids for Investigators. 7/87. Rockville, MD: DHHS, Office of Regulatory Affairs, Division of Field Investigations.

Chapter 9

Validation of a Device Manufacturing Facility with Multiple Product Lines

In a manufacturing facility that processes many products through the same production lines or equipment, the challenges of validation increase in complexity. A product-by-product approach to validation is no longer appropriate. One process validation event begins to impact another, and the work becomes redundant and inefficient. Suddenly, it becomes difficult to manage validation commitments with only the tools of process and product validation protocols.

Instead, a systems approach must be adopted that focuses on the validation of the **facility** to support a range of product processing events. The facility, in this case, is qualified for use; utility systems and clean rooms are validated; test methods common to many processes are validated; employees are trained; processing equipment is qualified (IQ and OQ); and then, as each new product is introduced into the facility, product-specific validations are performed to confirm that the facility and the processing equipment can support this new product.

A systems approach to facility qualification and validation requires a different level of planning than that described in the previous chapter. Commonly, a Facility Qualification Plan is written to describe the overall approach to GMP compliance and validation. This plan is supported by other major commitment documents, such as a Validation Master Plan. The purpose of these documents is to guide the decision-making process and record the decisions concerning how compliance commitments will be met in the corporation.

Technically, these documents are not a requirement of the FDA. Nevertheless, an inspector is likely to ask for them and, if they are not available, the inspector will ask for the information they are likely to contain.

Facility-based vs. Product-based Validation

There are validation events that are facility based and validation events that are product specific. In a facility that manufactures many products, understanding these divisions is essential when designing a validation program that is both efficient and effective.

Facility-based validations include utility systems (HVAC, compressed air or gases, house steam, clean steam, purified water, water for injection, clean rooms, chilled water, waste treatment), processing equipment (curing ovens, sterilizers, aseptic assembly lines, packaging equipment), test equipment, test stations, and monitoring/control software.

Utility systems in some device manufacturing facilities produce critical raw material components for final product processing. Purified water, clean steam, and compressed air that comes in direct contact with an implantable or invasive final product may, for example, have quality requirements that parallel those common for drug and biologic manufacturers. Power conditioning may be critical for a manufacturer of active devices. Clean room and controlled areas may be considered critical for implantable device manufacturers. Consider the impact of facility utility systems on your products and the need for validation.

The failure of processing or test equipment that could adversely affect the safety, uniformity, reliability, or performance of final product must also be considered for validation. If the equipment is used for many products, then it may be more efficient to validate the processing equipment as a part of the facility, establishing that it can perform reliably and reproducibly within the range of operation applicable to all products.

The validation of facility-based systems does not eliminate the need for product-specific validation, but it can simplify the event. If a new product is introduced into a facility with validated utilities, validated processing, and validated test equipment, then the validation of the product simply confirms that product specifications fall within the existing limits and that the processing steps can be performed reliably and reproducibly. (See chapter 8.)

The Facility Qualification Plan

The Facility Qualification Plan describes the compliance commitments of the corporation and how those commitments will be fulfilled and/or supported by the organization. This document is a primary document and, therefore, provides a map to all other documents in the facility's documentation system. If a Quality Manual is a requirement of your corporation, then it contains or references the information relating to all facility issues. Product-specific quality commitments are made and organized through other documents. An example format for a Facility Qualification Plan is in the appendix to this chapter.

The Validation Master Plan

In order to minimize the redundancy of testing and to use resources efficiently, validation must be planned as a system of interacting events. The Validation Master Plan defines the corporate commitment to validation and describes how that commitment will be met. This plan also assigns responsibility for validation. It is suggested that a validation team or committee be formed, made up of members from each department within the manufacturing facility. This validation team should be responsible for deciding what is validated and the level or extent of the evaluation. They should review and approve all validation protocols; they should review and approve all completed validation packages/reports.

The remainder of the Validation Master Plan should contain guidance and information that applies to all validation events. For example,

- Describe the types of validation that are appropriate to your operation (i.e., utilities, equipment, processing, software, etc.).

- Describe the levels of validation of options for evaluation.

- Provide guidance on how to make the decisions for how much evaluation is appropriate.

- Provide guidance on the format of the validation protocol.

- Provide for the use of amendments to validation protocols.

- Describe scheduling issues, as well as how to schedule validation events.

- Describe how deviations during validation will be handled.

- Describe the options for validation data handling, review, and approval.

- Provide guidance on revalidation.

- Describe the documentation requirements of validation.

- Provide reference to other, more specific guidance documents of equipment validation, process validation, software validation, as appropriate.

When a manufacturing facility is new, recently remodeled, or recently subject to validation requirements, the task of planning the validation of all equipment, methods, processes, and utility systems extends from the Validation Master Plan. The work plan must flow logically, beginning with utilities and processing equipment and culminating in product processing validation events.

Planning a facility-wide validation begins with listing the utility and environmental systems, processing equipment, test equipment, and software used for GMP manufacturing. Each list is then categorized into three levels of concern:

I. Systems that will be identified, calibrated, and maintained according to the routine monitoring and control programs of the corporation

II. Systems that will be qualified (i.e., IQ and OQ evaluations)

III. Systems, equipment, or software that will require validation (i.e., IQ, OQ, and PQ evaluations)

When the validation commitments of the corporation have been made, then the Validation Master Plan can be written; an example has been provided in the appendix to chapter 7. The Validation Master Plan usually references specific documents that describe how to write equipment and utility validation protocols, test method validation protocols, or process validation protocols. These documents are guidance documents that contain format requirements and content suggestions for each category of validation protocol. Examples are provided in the appendix to this chapter.

Chapter Appendices:
Facility Qualification Plan—An Example

1.0 The Business

Provide a brief history of the business. If this is a division of a larger company, a subsidiary, or another entity, declare this. Also mention whether it is a privately held or public corporation. Cite the corporation name changes that may have occurred over the years. Declare the purpose of this facility; be specific about the regulatory classification of products it is designed to support.

2.0 The Commitment

Provide a statement about the corporate commitment to GMP, international standards, EC Directive Essential Requirements, and other principles of operation that will apply to this facility.

3.0 The Manufacturing Facility

Describe the purpose of the facility (i.e., what it has been designed to do in the product manufacturing process).

3.1 Building Layout

Provide a floor plan of the building, indicating room numbers and departmental and dedicated processing areas. Indicate major containment areas and/or the boundaries of different air handling systems.

3.2 Flow of Materials, Personnel, Product, Waste, and Air

Provide facility floor plans that describe the flow of material, personnel, product, waste, and air (pressurization).

3.3 Major Utility Systems

List/describe the major utility systems that support GMP manufacturing in the facility (e.g., conditioned electricity, compressed air, purified water, water for injection, house steam, clean steam, HVAC, chilled water, and clean room areas).

3.4 Major Product Process Equipment and/or Systems

List/describe the major product processing systems or lines in the facility that are supported by equipment (e.g., injection molding, automated assembly, automated inspection, packaging, drying, curing, aseptic filling, and lyophilization).

3.5 Test Equipment

List/describe the major equipment used in the laboratory to test raw material components, processing intermediates, subassemblies, or final product (e.g., tensile tester, HPLC, and IR spectrophotometers).

3.6 Automated Processing

List automated processing events used in the facility to control, monitor, or record information about equipment or operations. Indicate whether the controlling software is purchased or developed in-house.

4.0 Departmental Organization

Provide an organizational chart of reporting structures in the manufacturing facility, as well as the number of employees in each area.

5.0 Master Validation Plan

Describe the commitments to validation for processing equipment and utility systems, test/inspection methods, device software, GMP software, and processing that is not already described in product-specific manufacturing plans. The Master Validation Plan is usually a separate document that is simply referenced in this plan.

6.0 Monitoring and Control Systems Plan

Describe the programs for monitoring and controlling operations within the GMP manufacturing facility, and provide specific references to document numbers for these programs. For example,

- GMP training of personnel
- Cleaning and disinfection programs
- Environmental monitoring and control programs
- Material movement and control programs
- Production process control programs

- Electrostatic discharge control programs
- Vendor certification programs
- Preventive maintenance programs
- Calibration and metrology programs
- QA investigation programs
- Quality assurance audit programs

7.0 Documentation System Plan

Describe the general principles of GMP documentation for the facility and the individual components of the documentation system (i.e., part number, specifications, SOPs, lot numbers, and work orders). General categories of documents include commitment documents, directive documents, and data collection documents. Reference specific documents about format, content, review, approval, distribution, filing, archiving, and change control.

8.0 Change Control Quality Plan

Provide a commitment to change control (i.e., that management recognizes that major changes in the business, the facility, personnel, or products could impact the GMP acceptability of this facility). Commit to auditing this plan, as appropriate, or at least annually to assess the impact of any changes. Reference programs for the detection of change, the prevention of change, and the control of change (i.e., evaluation and investigation of change and documentation change control).

In facilities that campaign products, it would be appropriate to discuss product changeover policy and procedures.

9.0 Facility Qualification Acceptance Criteria

Describe what commitments must be fulfilled (i.e., completed, reviewed, and approved) before the facility is considered GMP compliant by management. This approval should be in writing.

Equipment and Utility Validation Master Plan— An Example

1.0 Purpose

This GMP document extends the commitment to validation described in Facility Qualification Plan by providing guidelines for designing equipment or utility system validation protocols.

2.0 Scope

These practices apply to all equipment and utility systems validated to support routine GMP processing of product for human or commercial use.

3.0 Responsibility

The design of a validation protocol for equipment or utility systems is the responsibility of the validation committee.

4.0 Practices

Equipment/utility validations require three phases of evaluation, known as **qualifications:** installation qualification (IQ), operational qualification (OQ), and performance qualification (PQ). A validation is complete only when all three qualification events have been completed and are acceptable.

4.1 Installation Qualification (IQ)

The validation of a piece of equipment or a utility system begins with an installation qualification. The IQ study should establish confidence that the equipment or utility system is properly and safely installed. This means that the physical/structural installation meets the manu-facturer's suggested guidelines and that all utility support systems—electric, gas, steam, compressed air, and water—meet design limits and codes.

Installation qualification studies must be documented. A typical IQ document lists installation specifications and provides a signature block for maintenance to assure, by signature, that the equipment installation requirements and specifications are met and will continue to be met. The IQ document contains the following information:

- **Equipment identification information:** Provide the equipment identification numbers, the manufacturer's model and serial numbers, equipment size, dimensions, weight, capacity, and location (room number) in the facility. Include references to blueprint and drawing numbers, when appropriate.

- **Equipment utility requirements:** Describe services such as water, electric, gas, compressed air, steam, nitrogen, drain, and exhaust lines. Indicate the quality of feed utilities and any quantity or volume requirements. Similarly, indicate piping requirements (e.g., pipe composition, diameter, filters, reducers, etc.).

- **Equipment safety features:** Describe pressure relief valves and alarms and the settings at which they will be triggered. Other potential safety requirements include room temperatures, discharge-line sizing, alignments, and sound proofing.

- **Software:** If the equipment is operated by software, consult GMP XX on Software Validation Guidelines.

4.2 Operational Qualification (OQ)

When the installation of equipment is acceptable and the IQ document has been completed and approved, an operational qualification (OQ) is initiated. An OQ study establishes that the equipment can operate within established limits and tolerances. This demonstration of basic equipment performance must involve all operational aspects of the equipment that will be used routinely in manufacturing.

In the OQ section of the validation protocol, describe the calibration requirements for any measuring devices on the equipment or utility systems. Describe equipment cleaning requirements, pressure tests, or passivation requirements. Describe how to test the equipment system to ensure that it performs its intended functions consistently and reliably under ideal conditions. The protocol should include the following sections:

- **Calibration requirements:** Indicate the parameters, how they will be measured or monitored, and what is considered an acceptable range or limit. Include critical measuring and monitoring devices such as timers, pressure indicators, flow meters, temperature sensors, and any chart recorders that document performance. If a sensor performs a controlling function within the unit, describe how this control is achieved and/or monitored throughout a cycle.

- **Preoperational activities:** Describe tasks unique to initial start-up, as well as those appropriate for annual or periodic qualifications. Such activities include cleaning and sanitization of piping systems, passivation of stainless steel tanks and/or distribution lines, and software checks. In addition, it may be appropriate to check such things as door gasket integrity, vibration of blowers and motors, door interlock functions, cycle set points, and the performance of all heating elements.

- **Operations:** Describe how to exercise all electromechanical options on the equipment and provide performance acceptance criteria.

- **Acceptance criteria:** Describe an acceptable outcome for all tests conducted during the OQ. At the conclusion of this phase of testing—and before proceeding to the performance qualification—the data must be reviewed and a written declaration issued stating that results are acceptable.

4.3   Performance Qualification (PQ)

Once it has been established that the equipment is properly installed (IQ) and that it functions within specified operating parameters (OQ), it must be demonstrated that it can perform reliably and reproducibly under worst-case conditions.

Performance should be demonstrated with product under routine operating conditions. Worst-case conditions can be demonstrated by assuring that all ideal processing parameters, defined during the OQ, are met with maximum loads or capacities.

For utility systems such as WFI or steam, the PQ can demonstrate the production of acceptable quality water or steam during three cold starts at all points in the system. Worst-case conditions for utility systems, however, are best evaluated over time with rigorous monitoring programs, as it is only when filters fail, regeneration beds exhaust, or distillate columns begin to accumulate silica deposits that one can truly assess the worst case.

The PQ of a sterilizer should demonstrate that heat and/or steam, radiation, or gas penetrates into the materials in the chamber to effect sterilization. Effective sterilization is usually demonstrated by challenging the chamber load with a known bioburden and then demonstrating kill of this bioburden.

Over the years the worst-case approach for some applications has developed into a minimum/maximum load approach. This is because the minimum load will often demonstrate the worst case for some critical parameters.

Once the design of the process qualification has been established, the PQ section of an equipment validation protocol can be written. It should describe preliminary operations, performance qualification, and acceptance criteria.

- **Preliminary operations:** This section of a validation protocol includes the validation of biological indicators such as spore strips or endotoxin, the preparation of components to be sterilized, and the establishment of component loading configurations. All components used for validation work should be processed as they would be routinely.

- **Performance qualification procedures:** A PQ study should demonstrate that the equipment or utility system can consistently meet the operating specifications and perform its intended function (sterilization, depyrogenation, lyophilization) during at least three consecutive successful cycles.

  Before initiating a performance qualification, ensure that operating SOPs and processing forms accurately describe acceptable loading configurations and cycle parameters. Forms with a diagram of the empty chamber allow technicians to confirm, cycle-to-cycle, the location of materials and thermocouples in the chamber. Ensure that the processing of materials used in validation studies is equivalent to routine processing. Then run three consecutive cycles for each configuration and collect all recording charts, processing forms, and/or batch records for review.

- **Performance qualification acceptance criteria:** Ensure that all processing parameters meet the specifications cited in the validation protocol, that the raw data are available to support these claims, that all biological indicators test sterile, and that the number of consecutive runs meets requirements.

4.4   Validation Acceptance Criteria

When it is determined that the validation is complete and acceptable, the validation committee issues a certificate indicating the equipment number of the unit, the date validation was completed, reference to the validation protocol number and edition number, and an expiration date for the validation. This validation certificate is posted on or near the equipment.

4.5   Categorization of Equipment/Utility Validations

Equipment and utility systems should be categorized in order to determine how much evaluation is required to assure consistent, safe operation for its intended purpose. Full validations (IQ, OQ, PQ) will be required for equipment/utilities that are unique to your operation, equipment that is used in a manner other than that recommended by the manufacturer of the unit or for critical processing, or support equipment (sterilizers, lyophilizers, pure steam generators, etc.). Less rigorous evaluations may be appropriate for support equipment or utilities, for example, compressed air systems that only feed pneumatic controls. Less rigorous evaluation options include IQ only; IQ and OQ; or IQ, OQ, and an abbreviated PQ.

In determining the nature of an equipment or utility evaluation, consider the following questions:

- Does the utility or the performance of the equipment directly affect the safety, efficacy, or quality of the final product?

- What would be the impact of deviations or failure in these utilities or equipment?

- What is the likelihood that deviations or failures will occur?

- Can the utility/equipment be designed to prevent these failures? If not, is there any way to minimize the impact of failure?

Categorization requires good scientific sense and good business sense. It is used primarily to reduce the overall workload of validation while preserving the quality of the processing operations and the final product.

The final categorization of equipment is declared in the Equipment Validation Plan.

4.6   Validation Schedules

During the start-up of a facility and during annual revalidation activities, the order of equipment, utility, and process validation is important. Clearly, it would not make sense to validate an autoclave before the steam system that supplies the autoclave has been validated. Similarly, a pure steam generator should be validated after the WFI system. It usually follows that utility systems are validated prior to the initiation of equipment validation events and that all equipment and analytical methods are validated prior to the initiation of process validation events.

The validation schedule is also declared in the Validation Master Plan.

Test Method Validation Master Plan— An Example

1.0 Purpose

This document provides general guidelines for the format and content of a test method validation protocol. Guidance is also provided for determining the rigor of method qualification or validation activities based on the uniqueness of the analysis and/or its affect on final product quality, safety, efficacy, and stability.

2.0 Scope

These validation guidelines apply to all analytical testing performed on critical raw materials, processing intermediates, and final product manufactured at OLI.

3.0 Responsibility

Test method validation requirements will be determined by Quality Assurance. Test method validation activities will be performed by Quality Control and/or the department that routinely performs the analysis.

4.0 Protocol Introduction

Test method validation is required to determine the suitability of a given method to provide useful analytical data for a known set of samples. Analytical methods must be validated for specific uses. If instrumentation, reagents, or sample composition changes, revalidation may be required.

Once a Test Method Validation Plan is prepared, individual test method validation protocols can be written. The individual protocols provide detailed instructions about the number of replicates, sample composition/dilution, equipment calibrations, and so on.

4.1 Method Principles

This section describes the general principles at work in the analysis. Give a brief history of test method development, when appropriate. Also cite any known sample requirements or method sensitivities based on the principles of the method.

4.2   Method Suitability

Describe how the method will be used and why it is preferred to other test methods, when appropriate.

4.3   Method Categorization

There are many analytical methods performed in a Quality Control laboratory, and although all methods must be controlled, not all require a rigorous validation. As a result, methods should be categorized based on (1) their importance in assessing the critical identity, strength, stability, purity, safety, and efficacy parameters of products and/or (2) the uniqueness of the principles or techniques used in the analysis.

If, for example, a test method measures the potency of final product, it would be appropriate to fully validate the method. If, on the other hand, a method is an existing compendial method (heavy metals) or a generally accepted method (Biuret protein analysis), a less rigorous analysis may be sufficient; for example, a Level II method as discussed below.

There are three categories—Levels I, II, and III—as suggested by USP 23, Section 1225. Each category is tested as follows:

- **Level I tests** are analytical methods for the quantitation of major bulk components or active ingredients in finished product. Consider testing for

    precision
    accuracy
    selectivity
    linearity and range
    ruggedness

- **Level II tests (quantitative)** are analytical methods for testing impurities in bulk drugs or degradation products. Consider testing for

    precision
    accuracy
    limits of quantitation
    selectivity
    linearity and range
    ruggedness

- **Level II tests (limit tests)** are analytical methods for testing impurities in bulk drugs or degradation products. Consider testing for

accuracy*
limits of quantitation
selectivity
range*
ruggedness

- **Level III tests** are analytical methods used to determine performance characteristics of a drug or final product. Consider testing for

  precision
  accuracy*
  limits of quantitation*
  limits of detection*
  selectivity*
  linearity and range*
  ruggedness

4.4   Validation Procedures

4.4.1   Raw Material Control

The control of a test system depends directly on the quality and the control of raw material reagents. Review the reagents and components required to perform the test method. Ensure that part number specifications for these items adequately assess any critical parameters that would affect test method outcome. Review vendors for vendor-to-vendor inconsistencies. Change specifications as appropriate.

When reagents are prepared for test systems, declare or establish the stability of these reagents over time and in routine use conditions. Provide guidance about adequate storage conditions and expiration dates for these reagents.

4.4.2   Equipment Control/Calibration

The test procedure is also directly affected by equipment quality and equipment calibration/maintenance methods. Describe maintenance and calibration procedures for equipment used in the analysis. Refer to the appropriate SOPs.

---

* This evaluation may be necessary depending on the nature of the analysis.

In some cases full validation of the equipment may be required; in others a routine calibration record is sufficient. When routine equipment cleaning/adjustment/ calibration is required, either a logbook can be used to record events chronologically, or the information can be formatted directly into the test method data collection form.

In the case of HPLC columns that are used for more than one type of sample analysis, a chronology of use, regeneration, cleaning, and calibration must be kept. Also, procedures to evaluate column-to-column equivalency must be described/referenced.

4.4.3   Sample Acceptance Criteria

Sample volume, dilution, buffer components, pH, temperature, osmolarity, turbidity, and so on can also directly affect the performance of a test system. Indicate in the method validation protocol any sample-specific requirements. In addition, when appropriate, indicate a method for determining sample enhancement and inhibition of the testing method.

Any issues concerning the stability of samples should also be discussed. If samples are likely to change with time, provide guidance for test method performance within these time constraints.

4.4.4   Technician Training

Technicians must be trained specifically to perform analytical test methods; this training should be documented. The technician training program can be designed in conjunction with the ruggedness section of test method validation.

4.4.5   The Method SOP

Before initiating the validation of a method, ensure that the method SOP is written and that it accurately reflects the procedure as it will be performed. In addition, review the data collection form, assuring that all critical process control parameters will be recorded during validation procedures.

4.4.6 Method Evaluation

There are several aspects of an analytical method that can be evaluated. The following analytical performance characteristics should be considered when designing a method validation protocol. Each final protocol, however, will present individual method validation requirements according to an appropriate mix of the following performance characteristics.

4.4.6.1 Precision

Precision is a measure of test method reproducibility. Measure/evaluate the variation in homogeneous samples by performing several independent analyses and determining the mean, relative standard deviation, and coefficient of variance.

A minimum of five replicates with a relative standard deviation (RSD) of not more than (NMT) 2 percent is acceptable for most methods. The mean coefficient of variance should be NMT ±15 percent for samples at the middle and top of range; NMT ±20 percent would be acceptable for samples near the limit of quantitation.

4.4.6.2 Accuracy

Accuracy measures the compatibility of the test method value with a true or absolute value or standard. For example, demonstrate the ability of the test method to recover a known amount of analyte. This result is expressed as a percentage.

Replicates of at least five at concentrations near the limits of quantitation (LOQ) are required. At the middle and top of the acceptable range, recoveries/accuracies of 96–104 percent are acceptable; 60–110 percent are acceptable for concentrations below 100 ppb.

4.4.6.3 Limits of Detection

The limits of detection is the lowest concentration of a sample that can be detected with the method (not necessarily the lowest amount that can be quantified). Signal-to-noise ratios of 2:1 and 3:1 are generally acceptable.

When routinely performing the test, samples should contain 2–3 times the minimum amount capable of detection.

4.4.6.4 Limits of Quantitation

The LOQ is the lowest concentration of a sample that can be quantified with an acceptable degree of precision and accuracy.

For instrument methods determine the standard deviation of a series of blanks and multiply the standard deviation by 10 for an estimate of the LOQ. Confirm this with samples prepared at that concentration; use at least five independent standards.

4.4.6.5 Selectivity, Specificity, Interference

This is a measure of the method's sensitivity to impurities, related chemical compounds, and degradation products of product excipients. It measures the degree of interference.

Spike known concentrations of sample with known concentrations of potential contaminants and impurities. An RSD of NMT 2 percent is usually acceptable.

4.4.6.6 Linearity and Range

Linearity demonstrates that the method is capable of eliciting results that are mathematically related to the concentration of the analyte in the sample. Linearity is usually demonstrated over a defined range of analyte concentration, usually 5–8 points.

The slope of a regression line and its variance provide a mathematical measure of linearity; the y-intercept is a measure of potential method bias. Range is validated by demonstrating both accuracy and precision at its extremes.

If the test method relationship is not linear (i.e., log/log or log/linear), demonstrate these relationships as well.

4.4.6.7 Ruggedness

The ruggedness of a test method is a measure of its reproducibility in response to variations, such as different analysts, different instrumentation, different lots of reagent, and different elapsed test method times.

Compare the reproducibility of the test method when challenged under extreme conditions to the precision of the test method under normal conditions. For example, to evaluate the ruggedness of the test method when performed by different technicians, have four analysts perform one test per day for three days with identical samples and evaluate their precision.

Also evaluate the influence of freeze/thaw cycles on the test samples, standards, or reagents.

4.4.6.8 Correlation

If the test replaces an existing test method or is used to support another test method that measures a directly related characteristic, it may be appropriate to evaluate the correlation between methods. This evaluation will require that identical samples be tested several times by both methods.

4.4.7   Routine Monitoring of the Test Method

Each method validation procedure and each test procedure should indicate routine monitoring requirements, as appropriate. These requirements may include blanks, positive controls, negative controls, reagent testing, instrument readings, or calibrations.

These requirements allow for ongoing control of the procedure and assurance that the test method continues to meet validation criteria. Routine monitoring data can be used in audit activities for the method itself, for technician variability, reagent change evaluations, and the change in seasons.

4.4.8   Revalidation Requirements

The Quality Control or Quality Assurance Department can initiate a revalidation of a test method at any time. Significant changes in reagent vendors, instrumentation, and technicians could trigger a revalidation.

4.5   Test Method Validation Review, Approval, and Documentation Requirements

When an individual test method validation has been completed, compile the results into a report about the method. The report must be reviewed and the data checked for accuracy and completeness by at least two individuals, one of whom represents Quality Assurance. The reports should be filed in QA/Documentation.

Chapter 10

■■■■■■■

Validation at Vendors/ Subcontractors

It is common practice in medical device manufacturing to have several subcontractors interacting to produce final product. There are contract sterilization services for ethylene oxide and radiation sterilization of final products, contract testing laboratories, contract manufacturers of components or subassemblies, contract clinical testing organizations, contract installation and servicing, contract packaging, and contract distribution centers.

In order to assure quality in contracted manufacturing, the basic principles of quality assurance must apply to these relationships. This means that the quality of their operations or services must be established to meet expectations and requirements, including validation. Monitoring programs must be in place to routinely assess compliance in validated systems and processes. Changes to validated systems must be controlled; there must be evidence in the form of documentation to assure that all of these commitments have been met.

If suppliers, vendors, or subcontractors provide materials or perform operations whose quality could directly affect the safety, uniformity, reliability, or performance of the final product, then their manufacturing processes must also be candidates for validation. Validation is not something purchased from a contractor; it is a process that requires active participation. The quality of the validation event requires input from both sides. If subcontractors are chosen carefully, access to a valuable knowledge base will be gained. Ultimately, however, one must decide the appropriateness and extent of validation. This responsibility cannot be delegated.

Validation, however, is only one potential requirement of a contract relationship. Its success depends on the quality of the relationship as much as on the quality of the validation protocol. Validation events do not stand alone; they must be supported by programs that detect and control change. In this chapter we will review some fundamental requirements of a contract relationship as it applies to validation.

Who Is Responsible?

The client is responsible for the quality of its vendors and subcontractors. If process validation is required for a processing event that is performed by a subcontractor, then the client is responsible for the quality of that validation. Subcontractors are responsible for meeting standards and GMP requirements, but since the manufacturer is responsible for the safety, performance, and quality of the final product, the manufacturer "must do more than execute a business-only agreement with a contractor" (*Contract Sterilization Guidelines*/FDA). Do not assume, for example, that a contract sterilizer meets AAMI, ANSI, or ISO standards or the requirements of the FDA or the EC. Even if the subcontractor makes claims of compliance, assure that the standards and GMP requirements applicable to the manufacturer's product are met.

Validation at the Subcontractor

The subcontractor may have validated equipment and equipment systems for a wide range of operations to facilitate the many demands of various clients. If so, then review and audit this validation event and ensure that the operational parameters for your product are appropriate, that the test methods are appropriate, and that your processing requirements do not violate the existing validation.

If the existing validation is appropriate, then plan a performance qualification for your product in that system. No matter what the established evidence for validation, the subcontractor must demonstrate that with your product, the systems continue to operate reliably and reproducibly. Either the subcontractor or the client can draft a validation or qualification protocol. The client should retain copies of the protocol and the raw data package.

Managing the Contracts

Ensure that there is an individual with authority and responsibility in your corporation to monitor contract relationships. List the materials, processing, and services available for contract and who currently provides these materials or services. Categorize these materials/services into levels of concern; three levels should be sufficient.

The levels of concern should segregate the contract services into categories that will guide decision making about the rigor of evaluation necessary to assure the quality of the materials or services provided.

- **Category I:** Quality can be assured through incoming material or information inspection and testing. Occasionally, spiked samples or extra testing will be performed to assure vendor compliance with specifications.

- **Category II:** Quality can be assured with information supplied by the vendor; development samples and testing; and rigorous, routine inspection and test programs.

- **Category III:** Quality is assured through on-site audits and validation.

The decision making associated with Categories I, II, and III should consider the following:

- Is this a new vendor?

- Does the vendor routinely interact with clients in the medical products industry?

- What is the vendor's history of compliance?

- Does the vendor claim compliance with established QA systems (e.g., ISO, GMP, GLP)?

- Is the material or service provided unique?

- Is the processing required to produce the product or service unique?

- Is the equipment used in processing custom designed?

- Are the materials or information provided critical to the safety of your product?

- Are the materials or information provided critical to the performance of your product?

When designing a program to monitor the quality of subcontractors, provide for an adjustment in category designations based on history with the subcontractor. These changes in designation may occur because of excellent performance, resulting in a less rigorous testing schedule; or changes in designation may occur because of problems with subcontractors.

Changing Subcontractors

When changing subcontractors, the suitability of the new subcontractor must be demonstrated. At a minimum, the subcontractor must be qualified through a documented demonstration of equivalence between the new and old deliverables. In some cases, such as a change in sterilization facilities, this demonstration will involve revalidation.

If there is a biological or drug component in your device, changing the drug/biological substance manufacturer is likely to require new studies and validation work. This is because a different process usually results in a different product; a different manufacturing site, in itself, will result in different processing. Equivalence must be demonstrated.

Changing subcontractors may or may not have regulatory implications. For example, in the case of products approved through the Premarket Approval (PMA) process, changes in manufacturing facilities and methods require FDA review and approval prior to implementation if the changes affect the safety or effectiveness of the device. FDA review and approval is requested by submitting a PMA supplement. For other changes to PMA products, FDA notification at the time the requisite periodic reports are submitted may be sufficient. (Consult the PMA manual cited at the end of this chapter for more information.)

Changing subcontractors is a process that can be easily controlled if planned. Sometimes an unplanned subcontractor change is required because, for example, subcontractors may go out of business, may become victims of floods and fire, may be shut down by regulatory authorities, and may simply decide to discontinue a contract. Handling unplanned change is a difficult process; it is wise to consider backup subcontractors before a crisis occurs, especially for critical processes.

Chapter Appendix:
Points to Consider in Contract Relationships

Choosing a Subcontractor

It may seem obvious, but before you choose a subcontractor, ensure that they can

- Perform the work you will require,

- Meet appropriate standards and requirements,

- Perform required test methods,

- Support your operation as it scales up, and

- Perform validation studies, when appropriate.

Assuring the competency and adequacy of a subcontractor before the contract is written can be achieved in a variety of ways. If the subcontractor is a manufacturer subject to GMP requirements, ask to see their last FDA inspection report. This should consist of FDA Form 483: Inspectional Observations—a list of GMP concerns that the inspector leaves at the facility when the inspection is complete. When the inspector returns to his or her office, a narrative report is issued—the Establishment Inspection Report (EIR). If the subcontractor does not have copies of these items or refuses to share them, the information is available through the Freedom of Information Services (FDA, HFI-35, 5600 Fishers Lane, Rockville, MD 20857).

If a 483 citation notice has not been issued because there were no inspectional observations, there should be, at least, a Notice of Inspection, Form 482, and a summary EIR.

Visit the manufacturing or test facility. This can be an informal visit or a formal audit of operations. More information is gathered from this exercise than any other. Observe the operation and determine if the subcontractor is operating in a state of control. Consult the section on auditing later in this appendix.

The experience of others should be considered. Talk to other clients of this manufacturer, vendor, or testing laboratory; talk to those recommended by the manufacturer, as well as other clients, when appropriate.

If the subcontractor becomes, as a result of initial inquiries, a candidate for your business, it may be appropriate to have the subcontractor perform pilot studies or provide materials for testing. These materials can be used to assess the quality of the subcontractor's goods or services. This exercise also provides the subcontractor with a better understanding of the client's requirements and what it will take to perform the work properly. Ultimately, this will support the accuracy and completeness of the contract.

Establishing the Relationship

Establishing responsibility is fundamental to the quality assurance of the contracting relationship. This relationship is established with a contract or a written agreement, depending on the materials provided or services rendered by the subcontractor. For a subcontractor providing sterilization services for final product, the contract needs to cover both business issues and product-specific processing issues. Consider the following points when assigning responsibilities in a contract relationship:

- The duties of the contract
- The extent of duties
- Scheduling of work
- Length of contract
- Standards or regulatory requirements to be met
- Information transfer and primary contacts
- Termination of the agreement
- Confidentiality requirements

Product- or process-specific requirements can be written as amendments to the general contract. In this way, as new products come on-line, the requirements can be provided without any need to change the original contract. Product-specific instructions include the following:

- Sample or product identification requirements
- Shipping and handling requirements
- Storage requirements
- Loading configurations, cycle parameters and limits, and so on

- Process testing and monitoring requirements

- Employee training requirements

- Environmental controls and monitoring commitments

- Equipment calibration and preventive maintenance requirements

- Validation requirements for software, test methods, test equipment, and manufacturing

- Equipment, manufacturing processes, support processes, and so on

- Data collection and reporting requirements

- Reprocessing or rework guidelines

For a complex manufacturing event the device manufacturing or batch record is an extension of the contract. If properly formatted, the device manufacturing record makes all important commitments to the manufacturing event, such as an approved bill of materials, assembly instructions, sampling points, test points, acceptance criteria, equipment identification, and so on. The master record is signed by both the subcontractor and the client; it is the approved manufacturing process. A copy of this master record is generated for each manufacturing event. If changes are required, then a new record is issued and new signatures are obtained from both parties.

Other Contract Issues: When Things Go Wrong

The most important part of a contract is what will happen when things go wrong. Product may arrive after a scheduled date; a cycle may not run properly; test data may indicate unacceptable results. When things go wrong for known reasons, monetary penalties can be described in the contract. When things go wrong for unknown reasons, an accepted method of arbitration needs to be established. Insurance for "acts of nature" may be appropriate.

Quality Assurance: Remote Control

When the contract is established and product begins to move to and from the subcontractor, what assurances are in place to detect deviations from the contract and/or changes in the product or its processing? Ensure that the documentation is detailed and specific, indicating that critical parameters were tested and limits met for each event. Ensure that change is controlled. This is best assessed through periodic audits of the contractor.

Change Control with Vendors and Contractors

Given that the detection and control of change is difficult to achieve in your own organization, it is more difficult to achieve at a distance. This is because the client is removed from the decision making involved in change control at the subcontractor and because the subcontractor is not likely to understand the potential impact of change on client products.

Occasionally, what a vendor considers a product improvement has an adverse affect on a client's product. The only action that can reduce the likelihood of this happening is to communicate to the subcontractor what attributes of their product or processing are most critical to your product.

Documentation

Establishing what will be required, where the original records will be stored, and who will have access to them is a fundamental requirement in a contract relationship. In particular, what will happen to records if the subcontractor is either purchased by another company (potentially a competitor of yours) or the subcontractor ceases to exist?

The Audit

Auditing a subcontractor is the best way to collect the information that will support decision making about the relationship. Auditing, even in the best of relationships, is a necessary exercise designed to confirm the fulfillment of commitments and expectations.

The purpose of an audit is to establish confidence in a relationship that will rely routinely on verbal and written communication. In order to judge whether or not a subcontractor honors its written and verbal commitments, audit the subcontractor against existing commitments (i.e., against the existing or potential contract, against existing standards and regulatory requirements, against its own corporate commitments as described in corporate policy documents and procedures).

If appropriate, audit for GMP compliance. Consider the following:

- Is the facility generally clean and orderly? Is there adequate space to do the work? Do the employees seem knowledgeable about their work? Is staffing adequate?

- Are the utility systems that support production capable of producing quality materials consistently? Is the equipment properly calibrated and maintained?

- What is the potential for mix-up of products? What is the potential for cross-contamination between products or between different processing steps of the same product?

- What are the subcontractor's methods? How is contracted work documented and how are results reported? Are the methods appropriate? Are they followed? Is the data recorded clearly, is it reviewed and approved before it is released to the customer?

- How does the subcontractor handle samples or product? Is there sufficient control to prevent mix-ups? Are materials properly identified and stored in a suitable location?

- How does the subcontractor record and resolve complaints? How are out-of-specification results handled? How are investigations conducted? How are clients informed?

- How does the subcontractor release product? Is data reviewed for accuracy and completeness?

- What services/methods are contracted out? Who is used? What are the results of subcontract auditing?

Master Files

The master file is a vehicle of communication between a subcontractor and the FDA that may or may not be pertinent to a contracting relationship. There are five types of master files in the United States:

1. Type I, for manufacturing sites, operations, and personnel

2. Type II, for drug substances or intermediates, for device components or subassemblies

3. Type III, for packaging materials

4. Type IV, for drug components such as excipients or flavors for contract packaging or other contract manufacturers

5. Type V, for FDA-accepted information

A potential subcontractor may or may not have a master file with the FDA. If it does, obtain a copy of a letter of authorization from the company to the FDA authorizing access to their master file on behalf of your product. The letter should contain the master file number.

Current practice has discouraged the use of master files. The reviewers in Washington do not have easy access to these files and will usually ask for more information from the sponsor rather than dig through a master file. Given that it is good business practice to make a regulatory submission as convenient as possible for the reviewer, it is suggested that information about subcontractors be included in the submission whenever possible. This could be in a series of appendices. The only situation where this would not be possible is when a master file has been submitted to the agency to protect proprietary information.

References

Cady, W. W. 1992. PMA Applications: Manufacturing Section. *Regulatory Affairs,* 4:411–422.

Contract Sterilization Guidelines. FDA/CDRH.

Deciding When to Submit a 510(k) for Change to an Existing Device. FDA, CDRH Draft Guidance (April 8, 1994); available from the Division of Small Manufacturer's Assistance (DSMA), 800-638-2041.

Guideline for Drug Master Files. FDA/CDER, September, 1989.

Hinman, D. J., and N. J. Chew. 1990. Master Files: Streamlining Your Submissions, Protecting Your Secrets. *BioPharm,* March:12–18.

Kyper, Charles and Barcome, A. 1993. *Premarket Approval (PMA) Manual.* HHS Publication FDA 93-4214, April:I-13,14.

Lee, J. Y. 1990. Product Annual Review. *Pharmaceutical Technology,* April:86–92.

MAF Guideline (Draft). Regulatory Watchdog Service, Request #30467.

PDA Task Force. 1989. Supplier Certification—A Model Program. *Journal of Parenteral Science and Technology,* July:151–157.

PMA Manual, Part III. 4/93. FDA/CDRH, Publication #93-4214.

Tetzlaff, R. F. 1993. Validation Issues for New Drug Development: Part III, Systematic Audit Techniques. *Pharmaceutical Technology,* January:80–88.

Van Buskirk, G. E. 1990. GMP Audits: Pay Now or Pay Later. *Medical Device and Diagnostic Industry,* July:54–58.

Vincent, L. 1986. Quality Audits: Getting the Most out of GMPs. *Medical Device and Diagnostic Industry,* October:54–57.

Chapter 11

─────────

Monitoring Programs That Support Validated Systems and Products

Change is inevitable; uncontrolled change can be dangerous. Controlling change is fundamental to Good Manufacturing Practices, Good Design Development Practices, and Good Market Surveillance Practices in the medical products industry. Change, however, can occur unexpectedly. There must be programs for detecting change and programs to evaluate the impact of change should it occur.

Unexpected change observed in a validated system or process indicates that the system or process is operating out of control. When a validated system or product no longer performs reliably or consistently, the validation is no longer valid. In order to assure the continued validity of a validation event, therefore, one must monitor for changes that occur after validation is complete and investigate the impact of change and the options for corrective actions when necessary.

Who Is Responsible?

The evaluation of unexpected change in validated systems, processes, and products and the response to that change should be directed, monitored, and reviewed by a multidisciplinary group of individuals. There should be guidelines established for the investigation of unexpected changes. This will help to assure consistency in the decision-making process used to determine the significance of change and the seriousness of its impact.

Change Detection Programs

Although a validation event provides a level of confidence for change in a system or process (i.e., ruggedness), one must establish monitoring and control programs to assure that the conditions of the validation event are met routinely. If, for example, a heat sealer has been validated for a given range of dwell time, pressure, and temperature, and these parameters must be controlled, ensure that calibrated sensors routinely monitor these data points for compliance. If change occurs in the equipment, its operation, or its ability to properly seal a product, then the monitoring program should detect these changes. If these processing limits are not met, the validation has been violated and there is no evidence to assure that the package is properly sealed.

Change detection programs must be available for events that occur outside the company as well as inside the company. These programs form the net to catch unexpected change and the format to introduce corrective actions or planned changes systematically.

Change detection programs common to a manufacturing facility include the following:

- Electrostatic discharge monitoring programs
- Specification testing and approval of incoming materials, subassemblies or intermediates, and final product
- Environmental monitoring programs
- Bioburden monitoring programs
- Internal audit programs and trend analysis
- QA preclearance of production events
- Out-of-specification results reporting systems
- Programs that assure the identification and controlled movement of materials
- Preventive maintenance programs

- Calibration programs

- GMP training programs

- Cleaning and disinfection programs

Unexpected information about changes in product safety and performance coming from the marketplace can also invalidate a validated system, process, or product. These changes in product safety and performance can occur because

- Something has changed in the manufacturing and testing procedures that slipped through undetected,

- These are unanticipated problems for which no controls or detection systems have been previously designed, or

- There is an unanticipated impact of product shipping, storage, or usage.

As a minimum, programs must be in place to support the documented processing of customer complaints, returned goods, and field experience reports from salespeople, clinicians, patients, distributors, and so on. In addition, the FDA expects there to be a comprehensive postmarket surveillance (PMS) program in place to support Class III products, injectables, invasives, and so on. These PMS programs will vary in their complexity according to product risks, product delivery systems, and frequency of product exposure to patient (single use, chronic, or implantable).

When change is detected from the field, there should be an investigation of this change to determine the seriousness of its impact and appropriate and reasonable corrective actions. Corrective action may require revalidation of the system, processes, or products.

Programs designed to detect change in the field include the following:

- Complaint and field experience reporting programs

- Postmarket surveillance programs

- Returned goods reporting programs

- Product shipping and distribution reporting programs

- External audit programs

- Vendor certification programs

- Product servicing

Unexpected Change from Vendors

Change may also occur when a vendor changes a component, chemical, processing event, subassembly, or intermediate that could invalidate a validated system, process, or product. If the client is not informed of these changes by the vendor, then either the

- Change is detected through incoming inspection and test programs,

- Impact of the change is observed as a change in the safety, reliability, or performance of final product, or

- Change goes undetected.

Changes can be introduced into packaging materials, for example, by the vendor, that go unnoticed by the manufacturer until they affect product quality. These changes can affect penetration of sterilants; or seal integrity due to changes in adhesives, pouch composition, or rubber formulations.

In order to minimize the impact of change introduced by vendors, change detection and control programs should be established to

- Ensure open communication in contract relationships with vendors and subcontractors; written agreements with suppliers must assure change notification,

- Audit vendors for compliance, and

- Periodically test critical components for their full range of specification testing, upon receipt or in process.

Change Control Programs

In a regulated industry significant changes, whether they are planned changes or corrective actions, are controlled by requiring review and approval before they are implemented. All changes to validated systems, processes, or products must be reviewed and approved before implementation.

Changes are usually implemented through a qualification or validation program, a change in documentation, employee or customer notification, and retraining. When appropriate, the FDA is notified prior to implementation.

When Preapproval from the FDA Is Required

21 CFR, Part 807.81, requires that a 510k submission be made if a device or component is new; significantly changed or modified; or if the intended use of the device component is new, significantly changed, or modified. This means that when a product is changed or an unexpected change is detected, the significance of the change must be determined. If it is significant, then revalidation may be required and the FDA may require notification before the change can be implemented. The FDA believes that the manufacturer is best qualified to make the judgment about the significance of change. Whatever the judgment, however, it must be documented.

> Some manufacturers with highly qualified personnel and substantial experience may feel confident in performing various technical operations and analyzing results to determine that a particular change in a device, component or manufacturing process will not significantly affect safety or effectiveness of the device. After technical activities are completed and documented, the results should be reviewed by a design-review panel, change control board or equivalent group. After reviewing changes, if you are confident because of your design evaluation, change control procedures, equipment qualification, equipment calibration, process validation, personnel training and routine manufacturing procedures—that the change(s) could not significantly affect safety or effectiveness of the device, then the intent of the regulation has been addressed and there is no need to make a regulatory submission such as a 510k, premarket notification. After thorough review of proposed changes, if a manufacturer is uncertain whether a change may significantly affect safety or effectiveness or believes that a change will significantly affect safety and effectiveness then a regulatory submission must be submitted. (*Device Manual,* chapter 7)

Significant change in any device will require a new 510k submission or a supplement to the PMA. These significant changes include but are not limited to all design changes intended to correct an unanticipated failure of a product requiring FDA notification, and any changes in a significant risk product that could affect safety and performance that will also require FDA notification.

There are codified, mandatory requirements for the notification of the FDA when deaths or injuries occur in association with the use of a product. This information comes to the corporation through change detection programs.

Changes That Occur During a Validation Event

Occasionally, a validation event does not "go as planned" (i.e., what seemed a reasonable specification cannot be met). An initial validation of a curing oven, for example, is expected to meet a temperature specification of ±5°C. Thermocouple data from runs, however, does not support this specification. A meeting of the material review committee concludes that the oven is not capable of meeting this specification and that the product will not be adversely affected by an 8°C range, which the oven is capable of supporting. What happens to the validation protocol and the supporting data?

The protocol should stand as written, but it can be amended to change the specification. This amendment process can occur, however, only if this mechanism of change has been established before the event requires it. The amendment process is usually established in the Validation Master Plan.

Revalidation

Revalidation is one option for action that results from change. Revalidation, however, just like initial validation, must be designed appropriately. If there is a change in packaging materials for a heat-sealed package, for example, it would be appropriate to revalidate the packaging event, but it would not necessarily be appropriate to repeat the IQ and the OQ of the unit.

Revalidation in this case might simply require a performance qualification of the new material, demonstrating that the new sealing process operates within previously validated sealing parameters of the equipment and that the new package can be sealed repeatedly and reliably. One might choose to challenge the event at the lowest heat setting for the shortest dwell time with minimum pressure and the thickest packaging material. That challenge would be complemented by trials at the highest temperature, longest dwell time, maximum pressure, and thinnest package. Similarly, if the software controller were changed on the same heat sealing unit, a full validation would probably be appropriate.

Revalidation will be discussed in the next chapter.

References

Ashar, B. 1991. Handling Complaints Systematically: The Right Approach. *Medical Device and Diagnostic Industry,* September: 53–56.

Bachmann, J. 1991. Seizing Control of Product Changes. *Medical Device and Diagnostic Industry,* November:44–48, 86–88.

Change Control. 1991. *Medical Device GMP Manual.* 5th ed. FDA/CDRH, FDA 91-4179.

Federal Court Interpretation of cGMPs on Test Failure Evaluations. 1993. *The Gold Sheet,* February:7–12.

Kahan, J. S. 1990. Clarifying FDA's Policy on Device Modifications. *Medical Device and Diagnostic Industry,* June:101–104, 205.

Morgan, J. W. 1991. Decision Dilemma: Product Changes and Field Activity. *Medical Device and Diagnostic Industry,* March.

Out of Specification Result Requires Lab Investigation. 1993. *The Gold Sheet,* February:1–6.

Sheridan, R. 1993. How to Manage Regulatory Submissions for Device Modifications. *Medical Device and Diagnostic Industry,* October:64–70.

USA vs. Barr Laboratories, Inc., U.S. District Court for the District of New Jersey, Civil Action #92-1744.

Chapter 12

Revalidation

Revalidation should be considered when change occurs to validated equipment, test methods, and manufacturing processes and/or when a preestablished amount of time has passed. There should be guidelines written to describe these corporate commitments to revalidation.

Evaluating Change in Validated Systems and Processes

Change can occur in validated systems. This change may be planned, as in upgrades of equipment components or improvements in system performance; or change may occur unexpectedly, as in equipment failure. All unexpected change to validated systems or processes must be investigated; all planned change to validated systems must be evaluated. One of the options for action resulting from either an investigation or an evaluation is revalidation.

Revalidation events should vary in their rigor according to the type of change and the potential impact of that change on the

- Safety of the product,
- Performance of the product,

- Uniformity of the product, or

- Safety and performance of the manufacturing equipment or process.

The Effects of Scale-Up in Manufacturing Processes

Changing the scale of an operation can be a significant change where revalidation may be appropriate. Scale-up may result in changes to

- Equipment systems used to process materials,

- Equipment surfaces (i.e., glass to stainless steel),

- Processing times that can result in changes in exposure times of the product to the environment,

- The storage times for raw materials or processing intermediates,

- The overall time required to manufacture a batch or lot of product,

- Personnel (i.e., changes in the number of personnel interacting with product or changes in the level of expertise of personnel), or

- The manufacturing site or changes in the location of processing within the facility.

Although change resulting from scale-up in a device manufacturing environment may seem subtle, its impact can still be significant. When production levels increase in a facility, staffing and space suddenly become inadequate. This GMP violation can affect the safety and quality of product. Scale-up issues were some of the contributing factors in the Shiley heart valve incident.

Changes in Packaging Materials

Changes in packaging materials may be significant and may require evaluation or revalidation. Changes in materials for sterilized products, for example, can significantly change the properties of the sterilization process. Ethylene oxide penetration could be compromised, new residues could be generated, or new component interactions could be produced. A change in the size of a label, for example, initially judged to have no affect on the safety or quality of the product, in fact can cover so much of the Tyvek® pouch that EtO penetration and, therefore, sterility can be compromised.

Site Changes

Changing the manufacturing site for the production of product or subassemblies is a common practice in the device industry. Similarly, it is common to have more than one vendor capable of performing a process or providing a subassembly. If these services, however, involve validated processing or equipment systems, the impact of manufacturing site changes must be assessed when they occur and the quality of processing at multiple sites must be correlated.

Different facilities mean different utility systems, different environmental conditions, different equipment, different flow of materials, different personnel, and often different practices of accountability and traceability of materials and documents. All of these differences are changes that could affect product safety and quality.

Personnel Changes

People matter. The quality and performance of your staff is integral to the quality and performance of your product. A change in personnel, therefore, must be a planned and controlled event. Personnel must be trained in GMPs appropriate to your facility and product line before they work with product. Similarly, any product-specific or technical training must be completed before they are allowed to work unsupervised.

A significant change that occurs when a product manufacturing event is transferred to another site or another facility is the change in personnel. Do not minimize its potential impact.

Time-based Requalification/Revalidation

Since subtle changes in systems or processes cannot always be detected by routine monitoring and control programs and the impact of planned change cannot always be predicted, many companies choose to revalidate or requalify critical systems and processes routinely. These requalification programs are usually scheduled annually or semiannually and coincide with major preventive maintenance and calibration requirements.

In these situations a full performance evaluation may not be required if the review of historical files is satisfactory and a single, challenged performance run is acceptable. Design revalidation programs with a rigor that is appropriate and reasonable.

When validations are time based, then it is appropriate to post an expiration date for the validation on the validated system or equipment. This expiration date is usually incorporated into the validation certificate.

How Much Testing Is Enough?

Revalidation activities do not always need to be as intensive as initial validation events. If there is a change in packaging materials for a heat-sealed package, for example, it would be appropriate to revalidate the packaging event, but it would not necessarily be appropriate to repeat the IQ and the OQ of the unit.

Revalidation in this case might simply require a performance qualification of the new material, demonstrating that the new sealing process operates within previously validated sealing parameters of the equipment and that the new package can be sealed repeatedly and reliably. One might choose to challenge the event at the lowest heat setting for the shortest dwell time with minimum pressure and the thickest packaging material. That challenge would be complemented by trials at the highest temperature, longest dwell time, maximum pressure, and thinnest package. Similarly, if the software controller were changed on the same heat sealing unit, a full validation would probably be appropriate.

Decision making will be discussed in appendix A.

Installation Qualification Protocol

When a revalidation event is scheduled, confirming that the current installation continues to meet the specifications of the original IQ document is a simple task. If no changes have occurred, a knowledgeable mechanic can review the system and sign off the new OQ document within minutes.

This revalidation event, however, offers the opportunity to schedule or perform several tasks that are both appropriate to this evaluation and cost-effective. First, the maintenance engineer should review the equipment history files (i.e., the file or files containing preventive maintenance records, calibration records, and work orders from unscheduled repair events. This review should be documented and should assess whether the history files accurately reflect the history of the equipment system or processing event. During this review the engineer should determine if

- The commitments to preventive maintenance have been met,

- The commitments to routine calibration have been met, and

- There were changes to the system or process since the last IQ event, if these changes were documented, and if the rationale for these changes continues to be appropriate and reasonable.

Operational Qualification Protocol

Although an OQ event can be performed without changing testing parameters or limits of operation, a revalidation event offers an opportunity to "tune the system" to operating specifications that are more appropriate and reasonable. It is assumed that "tuning the system" will result in changes that tighten specifications, rather than broadening them. Tightening limits can be done without investigation; changing the acceptance criteria to accept values that would have previously been out of specification, however, requires an investigation and, depending on the seriousness or impact of the change, may require preapproval from the FDA.

During the OQ phase of the revalidation event, one should confirm through evaluation and study that the operating parameters and their limits continue to be appropriate. This requires a review of processing files for information that can be used in trend analysis. If performed, this review should be documented; if changes are suggested, the rationale for changes should also be documented.

When the review of operational parameters has been completed and the operational specifications for the equipment system or process redefined, one can write a new protocol or change an existing validation protocol to reflect these changes.

Performance Qualification Protocol

If a performance qualification is required during a revalidation event, the performance qualification should demonstrate reproducibility and the effects of challenge to the system. In addition, over the years of system evaluation, one should assess any trends in the validation data.

Documentation Requirements

Revalidation, just like initial validation, must be a planned event. The protocol must be written before the work begins. This protocol must be approved and controlled.

Revalidation files, folders, or notebooks should be maintained in the same location and in the same manner as original validation work. Similarly, validation certificates should be issued when revalidation/requalification work is complete; expiration dates should be assigned if this is company policy.

Appendix A

Decision Making: Points to Consider

Decision making (i.e., deciding how much testing is enough) is fundamental to the design of validation programs, to the design of change detection control programs, and to the investigation of change. All changes do not require the same degree of evaluation; all validation events do not require the same rigor; all change detection programs do not require the same sampling plan. Instead, decisions must be made. How a company makes those decisions is fundamental to an effective and consistent change control policy.

Decision making is a process. The outcome of the process is a decision, but the quality of that decision is directly affected both by the quality of the raw materials of the process (i.e., the accuracy and completeness of information) and by the quality of the decision-making process itself. To assure quality in the decision-making process, the process must be systematic. To assure consistency of policy there must be consistency of decision making within the corporation. Quality and consistency is assured through training of the decision makers of the corporation and the documentation of decision-making guidelines.

Decision making associated with planned change focuses on the significance of the product and the seriousness of the impact that change will have. The outcome of the decision-making process will affect the amount of evaluation that will occur and whether or not the FDA will be notified before change is implemented.

Decision making associated with unexpected change focuses on risk assessment. The results of this risk assessment will affect the manufacturing process, product acceptance criteria, the notification of users or patients, and, ultimately, the reputation of the product and the company.

Raw Materials of the Decision Process

Data Integrity

Procedures must exist to assure the accuracy and completeness of data. This includes data derived from QC testing, as well as from production events. This includes data generated internally, as well as externally (e.g., clinical trials, market experience, outside contractors).

The first line of defense for assuring the accuracy and completeness of data is to make every individual responsible for the data that he or she collects or generates. All data should be reviewed by a supervisor or manager or other knowledgeable individual. Finally, all data should be either directly reviewed or audited by Quality Assurance.

The Significance of Change

What Kind of Product?

The significance of change is influenced by the type of product for which change is proposed (i.e., device, diagnostic, biologic, or drug). The device industry, for example, is accustomed to making changes quickly and easily. They consider their ability to change their products (also known as configuration management) essential to their ability to remain competitive. This minimalist approach to change control may be appropriate for Category I and Category II Products, but it is increasingly difficult to justify for Category III Products.

Similarly, in vitro diagnostic (IVD) manufacturers work to the same agenda of market competitiveness. Their products are judged primarily on performance standards rather than on safety standards; product changes can often be thoroughly evaluated with bench-top testing. This approach works well until there is a biological substance introduced into the diagnostic kit, for example, and what is considered a simple change in a device manufacturing environment might require FDA preapproval in a biological manufacturing environment.

Changes in drug manufacturing are judged differently than changes in biologic manufacturing primarily because there are more analytical techniques available to detect changes in chemical molecules than in biological molecules. This makes it possible to make processing changes in a chemical synthesis or isolation event and "see" if the final product chemical structure is altered. Without an equivalent ability to detect change in biological molecules with bench-top testing, changes in biological processing are often judged as significant changes.

What Kind of Product Delivery System?

Clearly, the product delivery system directly impacts the significance of change. A device can be implantable, invasive, in patient contact, or support/auxiliary equipment. A diagnostic can be injectable, in patient contact, in vitro, or for home use. Drugs and biologics can be implantable, injectable, inhalant, transdermal, topical, or tablets and other oral dosage forms.

What Is Being Changed?

Is the change to the final product? If so, is it a raw material of the final product, a processing change, or a final product specification change?

Is the change to a subassembly or bulk intermediate? If so, are the specifications changing? Are they tighter than before? Is there a change in vendor? Is the new material from the new vendor equivalent to the old material? Can it be thoroughly tested?

Is the change in an analytical test method? If so, is the data generated from the method indicative of product safety or effectiveness?

The Impact of Change

What Are the Known Consequences of Change?

The impact of change is either unknown or known. Testing is one tool that can elucidate the impact of change, but testing may lead to inconclusive results and leave the impact of change unknown.

Change evaluation should be performed with the same scientific rigor that product design development testing is conducted. Options include bench-top testing, simulations, animal models, and human clinical trials. The level of testing is directly associated with the significance of the change and the seriousness of its known or potential impact.

What Are the Potential Problems Associated with Change?

When impact is known, there are often potential problems associated with the impact that also must be considered in the decision-making process for change. Consider the following process for evaluating potential problems:

- Identify/list the problem specifically.

- Determine or propose the likelihood of occurrence.

- If the likelihood is high, determine if anything can be done to eliminate the potential problem.

- If not, can the problem be detected with current monitoring and control programs?

- If detection methods are in place, prepare actions to minimize the impact of problems when they occur.

What Else?

What Guidance or Precedent Is Available from the FDA?

There may be guidance available from the FDA on changes to your product. If so, consider these in your decision-making process. In addition, there may be information available through Freedom of Information Services on competitor product changes that may have required agency preapproval.

What Political Factors Have an Impact on This Change?

In addition to assessing the significance of change and the impact of changes on products or patients, one must also consider, with significant risk/serious impact changes, the political climate in which this change occurs. Will these changes arouse public comment? Is this a precedent-setting change for the agency? Are you operating under a warning letter or serious 483 citations? What is your competition?

Although these issues are difficult to quantify in a decision-making process, they do have influence. Clearly, a change can appear insignificant and low in impact and yet require preapproval by the FDA for political reasons.

The Decision-Making Process

Who Decides?

Push the responsibility for making decisions about change down the line of management as far as appropriate and possible! In the examples provided in appendix B under out-of-specification (OOS) results, the court supports the use of informal investigations at the departmental level for single-event OOS results.

Clearly, simple changes and the majority of changes should be made at the departmental level without the need for Quality Assurance review. This does not mean, however, that the changes go undocumented. All change must be documented and rationale provided. Ultimately, all change should be reviewed by Quality Assurance through audits or periodic change review.

There is often a need for an intermediate level of change review, involving QA but not the entire Change Review Board. This type of change often involves validated equipment or more than one department. If appropriate, include this option in change control programs.

How to Decide?

Decisions should be made based on the guidance offered above. Consider the significance of change, the impact of change, and the political climate. If useful, develop a rating system for each category with examples. Then use a matrix approach and scoring system to determine, for planned change, options for evaluation and agency notification; for unplanned change, determine options for product or process evaluation/change, as well as consumer/agency notification.

Appendix B

Change Control: Points to Consider

Controlling change is a fundamental requirement of any Quality Assurance system. In a medical manufacturing environment all planned change must be evaluated; all unexpected change must be investigated. Change control programs common to medical products manufacturing include the following:

- Document change control programs
- Out-of-specification investigation programs
- Field investigation programs
- Engineering/process change orders
- Product changeover in a campaign manufacturer

Change Detection

Program Format

Each of these programs must be documented. Change detection programs should describe what type of information will be gathered, what methods will be used to collect information and process data, and the commitment to monitoring (i.e., sample acceptance criteria, sampling sites, sampling frequency, sampling methods, sampling volume or size, sampling schedules, testing techniques, test equipment, and acceptance criteria).

Acceptance criteria, when appropriate, should be formatted into alert limits and action limits. If a monitoring event exceeds an action limit, the equipment or process affected should be shut down until an investigation is performed. As a result, alert limits should be set to warn of change long before action is required. If a clean room is classified for no more than 100 particles per cubic foot of air, for example, and routine monitoring in the area recovers less than 10 particles per cubic foot, then the action level would be 100 particles/cubic foot and the alert level could be 25 particles per cubic foot.

Out-of-Specification Results

The change detection programs listed above are designed to monitor equipment systems, processes, environments, and personnel for change. When change is detected, an established limit or specification has not been met during routine processing. The test result is called an out-of-specification (OOS) result. This term originated from a court decision, known as the Wolin decision, in the District Court of New Jersey in 1992. This decision has placed new emphasis on the detection and the characterization of change in the manufacturing environment.

According to the decision, an OOS event can result from three possible errors:

1. **Laboratory or production-line error:** failure of the technician, test equipment, testing standards, and so on—errors that do not directly affect the batch manufacturing process or the product.

2. **Nonprocess-related error:** failure that affects the batch manufacturing process and is caused by equipment failure, environmental failure, operator error, and so on.

3. **Process-related error:** failure that affects the manufacturing process but is NOT caused by operator error, equipment failure, and so on.

Evaluation of OOS Results

The guidance that comes from the Wolin decision suggests that every OOS result must be investigated. There are two mechanisms for investigation: informal and formal. Informal investigations are appropriate for single-event OOS results. The informal investigation can take place at the departmental level between the technician and the supervisor. The investigation should be documented and follow a written procedure that directs the review of test procedures, calculations, equipment performance, and the data record.

Formal investigations are required when there are multiple OOS results, when contamination is detected, when mix-ups occur, and when cause is unknown. A formal investigation must include individuals outside the department, such as Quality Assurance. The investigation must

- Document the reason for the investigation;

- Provide a summary of the event that led to the OOS result;

- Include data from further evaluations or retests, as appropriate;

- Include a historical review of change and other supporting test results on the batch when appropriate to the investigation;

- Declare the characterization of the OOS result according to the three options listed above;

- Declare corrective actions to save the batch and to prevent recurrences of the event;

- List other batches affected; and

- Declare the disposition of the batch and provide signatures to support the decision.

Formal investigations should be completed within 30 days of the event. There is also specific guidance in the Wolin decision on the options traditionally used for evaluation (i.e., retesting, resampling, reworking/reprocessing, and using outlier tests to invalidate OOS results).

Appendix C.1

Preproduction Quality Assurance Planning:

Recommendations for Medical Device Manufacturers

Prepared by the Office of Compliance and Surveillance
Center for Devices and Radiological Health
U.S. Food and Drug Administration
September 1989

1.0 Scope

This document describes recommended design practices applicable to medical devices and is intended to assist device manufacturers in planning and implementing a preproduction quality assurance program. The purpose is to provide a high degree of confidence that medical device designs are reliable, safe, and effective prior to releasing designs to production for routine manufacturing.

The extent to which these recommendations are implemented is left to the discretion of the manufacturer, and may involve a consideration of the risk a device would present to the user if it were unsafe or ineffective. Some of the recommendations may be excessive for devices that are simple in design and present no risk to the user should they fail. However, all medical device manufacturers are encouraged to use these recommendations, especially those manufacturers who have found it necessary to recall devices from the marketplace because of defects in the design of a component, subassembly, or the device itself. Likewise, manufacturers of life-sustaining, life-supporting, or implantable devices, particularly those who make electrical, electromechanical, or mechanical devices, are encouraged to examine these suggested practices to determine whether they are applicable to product development. Additionally, manufacturers who are committed to company-wide quality assurance programs to enhance product quality and productivity, and who wish to minimize the cost of these programs, should find all or some of these recommendations helpful in identifying the preproduction activities that FDA believes are important.

The practices described herein are applicable to the development of new designs as well as to the adaptation of existing designs to new or improved applications. The word "should" is used in the document in reference to practices and procedures which, though recommended, are nonmandatory.

2.0   Introduction

The design phase is the most important phase in the life cycle of a device. The inherent safety, effectiveness, and reliability of a device are established during this phase. No matter how carefully a device may be manufactured or how perfect the GMP program, this inherent safety and effectiveness cannot be improved except through design enhancement. Therefore, it is crucial that adequate controls be established and implemented during the design phase to assure that the safety, effectiveness and reliability of the device are optimally enhanced prior to manufacturing to assure that an acceptable quality level can be achieved during production. It is only through careful planning and management of the preproduction process that safety, effectiveness, and reliability can be established in a device.

A design deficiency can be very costly once a device design has been released to production and the device is manufactured and distributed. Costs may include not only replacement and redesign costs, with resulting modifications to manufacturing, procedures, retraining, etc. to enable manufacture of the modified device, but also liability costs and loss of customer faith in the product.

These recommendations were developed in part from documents identified in Appendix B—References. The cited references include military standards, documents developed by the National Aeronautics and Space Administration (NASA), voluntary standards, National Bureau of Standards (NBS) guidelines, and others. (Note: NBS is now the National Institute of Science and Technology.)

Analysis of recall and other adverse experience data available to FDA indicates that one of the major causes of device failures is deficient design. Examples are cited herein, not as an indictment of particular manufacturers or industries, but as an illustration of the advantages of implementing a preproduction quality assurance program. The examples used are from FDA's device recall records.

3.0   Preproduction Quality Assurance Program

All manufacturers of medical devices should establish and implement a program for assessing the reliability, safety, and effectiveness of device design prior to releasing the design to production and, ideally, this assessment should be made as the design is developed. The procedures for making these assessments should be defined in a formally established and documented preproduction quality assurance (PQA) program. Formal protocols should be developed and agreed upon for design verification and reliability assessment. The program should be sanctioned by upper management and should be considered a crucial part of each manufacturer's overall effort to produce only reliable, safe, and effective devices.

3.1 Organization

The organizational elements and authorities necessary to establish the PQA program, to execute program requirements, and to achieve program goals should be specified in formal documentation. Responsibility for implementing the overall program and each program element should also be formally assigned and documented.

An audit program should be established as a permanent part of the PQA, and audits should be conducted periodically throughout the preproduction life cycle phase to evaluate program implementation and effectiveness. The program should be updated as experience is gained and the need for improvement is noted.

Manufacturers should consider the following activities when developing the PQA program and implement those controls most appropriate for assuring the safety, effectiveness, and reliability of the device design.

3.2 Specifications

Prior to the design activity, the design concept should be defined or expressed in terms of its desired characteristics, such as physical, chemical, performance, etc. Acceptable ranges or limits should be provided for each characteristic to establish allowable variations and these should be expressed in terms that are readily measurable.[1]

Once these characteristics are agreed upon as those desired for the proposed device (i.e. the design aim), they should be translated into written design specifications. These preliminary specifications provide the details from which the design can be developed and controlled, as well as the means by which the design can be evaluated. Specifications should address, as applicable, performance characteristics, such as safety, durability/reliability, precision, stability and purity, necessary to fulfill the product's intended purpose. The expected use of the device, the user, and the user environment should be considered when establishing the design's physical configuration, performance, safety and effectiveness goals (for example, location of controls, displays, allowable leakage currents, use in the home, etc.). Specifications should be reviewed and evaluated by qualified personnel from appropriate organization elements, such as Marketing, R&D, Quality Assurance, Reliability, and Manufacturing.

3.2.1 System Compatibility

A device's compatibility with other devices in the intended operating system should be addressed early in the design phase, to the

---

1. For example, the pulse amplitude range for an external pacemaker could be established as 0.5 to 28 mA at an electrical load of 1000 ohms, and pulse duration could be 0.1 to 9.9 ms.

extent that compatibility is necessary to assure proper functioning of the *system;* examples include IV sets with infusion pumps, breathing circuits with ventilators, disposable electrodes with cardiac monitors. The full operating range of within-tolerance specifications for the mating devices(s) should be considered, not merely nominal values.[2]

3.2.2 Design Changes

Changes made to the specifications during R&D that are accepted as design changes should be documented and evaluated to assure that they accomplish the intended result and do not compromise safety and effectiveness. Manufacturers should not make unqualified, undocumented changes during preproduction clinical trials in response to suggestions or criticisms from clinicians. In the manufacturer's haste to satisfy the user, changes made without an evaluation of the overall effect on the device could result in improving one characteristic of the device while having an unforeseen adverse effect on another.

The documentation of changes made to a device as it is developed provides a complete history of the product design evolution and a means by which each design change can be reviewed. This documentation can be invaluable for conducting investigations of design deficiencies which may not be detected until after the finished device is in commercial distribution.

3.3 Design Review

Device design should progress through clearly defined and planned stages. For example, a new medical device could be designed in planned stages including concept, detail design, prototype, and pilot production. Each medical device manufacturer should establish and implement, as the cornerstone of the PQA program, an independent assessment or review of the design at each stage as the design matures to assure conformance to design

---

2. For example, a disposable blood tubing set was designed and manufactured by Company A for use with Company B's dialysis machine. The tubing was too rigid, such that when the air-embolism occlusion safety system on the dialysis machine was at its lowest within-specification force, the tubing would not necessarily occlude and air could be passed to the patient. The tubing occluded fully under the nominal occlusion force.

criteria and to identify design weaknesses. Some manufacturers may find it advantageous to consult with outside experts. The objective of design review is the early detection and remedy of design deficiencies. The earlier design review is initiated, the sooner problems can be identified and the less costly it will be to implement corrective action. The assessment should include a formal review of subsystems, including software (when applicable), components, packaging, labeling, and support documentation such as drawings, test specifications, and instructions. The extent and frequency of design review depends on the complexity and significance of the device studied. However, the assessment should extend beyond merely satisfying user requirements and always assure that safety and effectiveness goals are met.

A detailed, documented description of the design review program should be established, including organizational units involved, procedures used, flow diagrams of the process, identification of documentation required, a schedule, and a checklist[3] of variables to be considered and evaluated.

Reviews should be objective, unbiased examinations by appropriately trained personnel who include individuals other than those responsible for the design. For example, design review should be conducted by representatives of Manufacturing, Quality Assurance, Engineering, Marketing, Servicing, and Purchasing, as well as those responsible for R&D. Design review should, as applicable and at the appropriate stage, also include

---

3. For example, a design review checklist could include the following, with the review consisting of an evaluation of the design to assure that each checklist item, as applicable, was adequately addressed. Each manufacturer should construct a checklist that is appropriate for their device.
   - Physical characteristics and constraints
   - Regulatory and voluntary standards requirements
   - Safety needs of the user, need for failsafe characteristics
   - Producibility of the design
   - Functional and environmental requirements
   - Inspectability and testability of the design, test requirements
   - Permissible maximum and minimum tolerances
   - Acceptance criteria
   - Selection of components
   - Packaging requirements
   - Labeling, including warnings, identification, operation, and maintenance instructions
   - Shelf-life, storage, stability requirements
   - Possible misuse of the product that can be anticipated, elimination of human induced failures
   - Product serviceability/maintainability

those designated to conduct and monitor preclinical and clinical studies. Provisions should be prescribed for resolving differences of technical judgment. Review results should be well documented in report form and signed by designated individuals as complete and accurate. All changes made as a result of review findings should be documented. Reports should include conclusions and recommended followup and should be disseminated in a timely manner to appropriate organizational elements, including management.

When corrective action is required, the action should be appropriately monitored, with responsibility assigned to assure that a followup is properly conducted. Schedules should be established for completing corrective action. Quick fixes should be prohibited. These include adjustments that may allow the device to perform adequately for the moment but do not address the underlying cause. All design defects should be corrected in a manner that will assure the problem will not recur. Design reviews should, when determined appropriate, include failure mode effects analysis.

3.3.1 Failure Mode Effects Analysis

Failure mode effects analysis (FMEA) should be conducted at the beginning of the design effort and as part of each design review to identify potential design weaknesses. The primary purpose of FMEA is the early identification of potential design inadequacies that may adversely affect safety and performance. Identified inadequacies can then be eliminated or their effect (susceptibility) minimized through design correction or other means.

FMEA is conducted by identifying, through failure analysis techniques, significant failure modes that can occur, their effect on safety and effectiveness, and the probability of occurrence. When it is likely that a failure could adversely impact on safety or effectiveness, the design should be modified to eliminate or minimize the failure cause. For those potential failure modes that cannot be corrected through redesign effort, special controls such as labeling warnings, alarms, etc. should be provided.[4] FMEA should include

---

4. For example, one possible failure mode for an anesthesia machine could be a sticking valve. If a sticking valve could result in over- or under- delivery of the desired anesthesia gas, a failsafe feature should be incorporated into the design to prevent the wrong delivery, or, if this is impractical, a suitable alarm system should be included to alert the user in time to take corrective action.

an evaluation of possible human-induced failures or hazardous situations.[5, 6]

Each potential failure mode should be considered in light of its probability of occurrence and characterized as to the severity of its effect on reliability, safety, and effectiveness.

FMEA should be conducted in accordance with a written protocol, with results and recommendations documented and provided to the appropriate personnel in a timely manner. When design weaknesses are identified, consideration should be made of other distributed devices in which the design weakness may also exist.[7] Appropriate action should be taken as necessary to correct these design deficiencies.

Typically, two failure mode analysis techniques are used: (1) Fault Tree Analysis and (2) Failure Mode Effects Criticality Analysis.

3.3.1.1   Fault Tree Analysis

Fault tree analysis (FTA) is a deductive, "top-down" approach to failure mode analysis. First, a system failure or safety hazard is assumed, Next, through the use of detailed logic diagrams, basic component failures or events are simulated to determine if the hazard could actually occur. Once identified, computational techniques are used to analyze the basic defects, determine failure probabilities, and establish severity of effect levels. FTA is especially applicable to medical devices because human/device

---

5. For example, defibrillator battery packs were recalled because of an instance when the battery pack burst while being charged. The batteries were designed to be trickle charged, but the user charged the batteries using a rapid charge. The result was a rapid buildup of gas which could not be contained by the unvented batteries. If a warning label had been provided or the batteries vented, the incident probably would not have happened.

6. In another example, a microprocessor-controlled infusion pump required an EPROM change because of the possibility of over-infusion. It was determined that if the "volume remaining" was manually set to zero and the "flow rate" set to less than 1 ml/hr, the pump would deliver fluids at the previous flow rate setting which could be as high as 699 ml/hr.

7. For example, an anomaly that could result in an incorrect output was discovered in a microprocessor used in a blood analysis diagnostic device at the prototype testing stage. This same microprocessor was used in other diagnostic machines already in commercial distribution. A review should have been made of the application of the microprocessor in the already-distributed devices to assure that the anomaly would not adversely affect performance.

interfaces can be taken into consideration, i.e., a particular kind of adverse effect on a user such as electrical shock can be assumed. Whether or not the event can occur, either because of a defective device or operator error, can then be determined.

3.3.1.2   Failure Mode Effects Criticality Analysis

Failure mode effects criticality analysis (FMECA) is an inductive "bottom-up" process which assumes basic defects at the component level and then determines the effects on higher levels of assembly. Failure modes are analytically induced into each component and failure effects are evaluated and noted, including severity and probability of occurrence. FMECA can be performed using either actual failure data derived from field failures or hypothesized failure modes derived from design analysis or other sources. In addition to providing information about failure cause and effect, FMECA provides a structured method for proceeding component-by-component through the system to assess failure effects.

FMECA is described in MIL-STD-1629A, "Procedures for Performing Failure Mode, Effects, and Criticality Analysis," and on-site training is offered by private firms.

3.4 Reliability Assessment

When appropriate and applicable, a reliability assessment should be made for new and modified designs and acceptable failure rates established. Reliability assessment is the process of prediction and demonstration directed towards estimating the basic reliability of a device. The appropriateness and extent of a reliability assessment should be determined by the risk the device presents to the user should it fail or become defective.

Prior to distribution, reliability assessment may be initiated by theoretical and statistical methods by first determining the reliability of each component, then progressing upward, establishing the reliability of each subassembly and assembly, until the reliability of the entire device or device system is established.[8] This approach,

---

8. For example, the following references apply to predicting the reliability of electronic devices:

a) MIL-HDBK-217B Reliability Prediction of Electronic Equipment

b) MIL-STD-785B Reliability Program for Systems and Equipment Development and Production.

c) Study of Reliability Prediction Techniques for Conceptional Phases of Development, RADC-TR-74-235, Rome Air Development Center.

however, provides only an estimate of reliability, since it does not simulate the actual effect of interaction of system parts and the environment. To properly estimate reliability, complete devices and device systems should be tested under simulated use conditions. The most meaningful reliability data are usually obtained from actual use.

The process of reliability assessment goes beyond merely making a prediction, testing, and then waiting for field experience to prove or disprove the assessment. Reliability assessment is a continuous process that includes predicting, demonstrating reliability, analyzing data, then re-predicting, re-demonstrating reliability, and re-analyzing data on a continual basis. Reliability assessment should be considered an essential part of the PQA program and should be used to estimate and establish the reliability of each new and modified design, when applicable.

3.5 Parts and Materials Quality Assurance

All medical device manufacturers should establish and implement a comprehensive parts and materials (P/M) quality assurance program for assuring that all P/M used in device designs have the reliability necessary to achieve their intended purposes. For some this can be done in-house, while for others it may be necessary to contract with suppliers or outside test labs. The reliability goal should be based on the severity of use and importance of the P/M function.[9] The P/M program should encompass the selection, specification, qualification and ongoing verification of P/M quality, whether fabricated in-house or provided by vendors. P/M quality assurance should include qualification of suppliers to aid in assuring only quality P/M are used.

P/M should be selected on the basis of their suitability for the chosen application, compatibility with other P/M and the environment, and proven reliability. Conservative choices in selection of

---

9. For example, the spring used to achieve proper spindle operation in a volume ventilator experiences thousands of cycles of compression and expansion, and failure of the spring could result in respiratory arrest. Therefore, the spring's ability to perform reliably under these conditions must be assured through comprehensive qualification testing. Operator and service manuals should cover appropriate preventive maintenance.

P/M are characteristic of reliable devices. Standard proven P/M should be used as much as possible in lieu of "unproven" P/M.[10]

A preferred P/M list should be established during the preliminary design stage and refined as the design progresses. This list should include approved suppliers for the P/M and be placed under formal change control once the design is released for production. P/M should be classified according to the severity of their effect on reliability, safety, and effectiveness should they fail or not achieve their intended purpose. Emphasis on the use of high reliability P/M, qualification, inspection, test, and other methods of assuring acceptability should be based on this classification; i.e., more emphasis should be placed on assuring the acceptability of P/M whose failure could result in injury.

The acceptability of P/M for their selected applications should be determined and supported by both calculated and observed test data. Proper application means not only assuring P/M will perform but that they are not unduly stressed mechanically, electrically, environmentally, etc.[11] A thorough applications review should be conducted during the design phase and, when necessary, adequate margins of safety should be established. Existing test or qualification data may be used for proven or standard P/M. However, when selecting P/M previously qualified, attention should be given to whether the data are current, the applicability of the previous qualification to the intended application, and the adequacy of the existing P/M specification. Additional qualification should be conducted as necessary.[12]

---

10. For example, a manufacturer of an intravenous administration set used an unproven plastic raw material in the initial production of molded connectors. After distribution, reports were received of the tubing separating from the connectors. Investigation and analysis by the manufacturer revealed that the unproven plastic material used to mold the connectors deteriorated with time, causing a loss of bond strength. The devices were subsequently recalled.
11. For example, a whole-body imaging device was recalled because screws used to hold the upper detector head sheared off, allowing the detector head to fall to its lowest position. The screws were well within their tolerances for all specified attributes. However, the application was such that the screws did not possess sufficient shear strength for the intended use.
12. For example, lubricant seals previously qualified for use in an anesthesia gas circuit containing one anesthesia gas may not be compatible with another gas. These components should be qualified for each specific environment.

Failure of P/M during qualification to meet expected performance, safety, and effectiveness objectives should be investigated and the results described in written reports. These reports should be provided to management and other appropriate personnel in a timely manner to assure that only qualified P/M are used. Failure analysis, when deemed appropriate, should be conducted to a level such that the failure mechanism can be identified.

3.6 Software Quality Assurance

When a design incorporates software developed in-house, a software quality assurance program should be in place that outlines a systematic approach to software development. The program should include a protocol for formal review and validation of device software to ensure overall functional reliability.

There are many approaches to software quality assurance (SQA), and some of these are described in the software source documents referenced at the end of this document. However, they all involve some form of measuring the development process at each phase; for example, establishing requirements, validating that the output of each phase satisfies its requirements (which may include testing), documenting and controlling changes that are made, and revalidating. Major goals of SQA are correctness, reliability, testability, and maintainability.

SQA should begin with a plan, which can be written using a guide such as ANSI/IEEE Standard 730-1984, IEEE Standard for Software Quality Assurance Plans. Good SQA assures quality software from the beginning of the development cycle by specifying up front the required quality attributes of the completed software and the acceptance testing to be performed. In addition, the software should be written in conformance with a company standard using structured programming. The SQA representative or department should have the authority to enforce implementation of SQA policies and recommendations.

When device manufacturers purchase custom software from contractors, the SQA should assure that the contractors have an adequate SQA program that will assure software correctness, reliability, testability, and maintainability.

When manufacturers purchase "off-the-shelf" software from vendors or subcontractors, the SQA should assure, through appropriate testing, that the software is adequate for its intended application prior to use in production.

3.7 Labeling

A review of labeling should be included as part of the design review process to assure that it is in compliance with applicable laws and regulations and that adequate directions for the product's intended use are easily understood by the end-user group. Labeling includes manuals, charts, inserts, panels, display labels, recommended test and calibration protocols, software for CRT displays, etc. Qualification testing of the device should include verification of the accuracy of instructions contained in the labeling.[13] Qualification should also include verification that labeling intended to be permanently attached to the device will remain attached and legible through processing, storage, and handling for the useful life of the device.

Maintenance manuals should be provided where applicable and should provide adequate instructions whereby a user or service activity can maintain the device in a safe and effective condition.

3.8 Design Transfer

Once the design is translated into physical form, its technical adequacy, safety and reliability should be verified through comprehensive documented testing under simulated or actual use conditions.[14]

Clinical trials should not begin until the safety of the device has been verified under simulated use conditions, particularly at the expected performance limits. Simulated use testing should address use with other applicable devices and possible misuse. Manufacturers of devices that are likely to be used in a home environment and operated by persons with a minimum of training and experience should anticipate the types of operator errors most

---

13. For example, after distribution, labeling had to be corrected for an infusion pump because there was danger of over-infusion if certain flow charts were used. The problem existed because an error was introduced in the charts when the calculated flow rates were transposed onto flow charts.

14. For example, an infusion pump was recalled because of over-infusion. Investigation revealed that there was a compatibility problem between the pump and IV set cassettes. The receptacle valve actuating stud was too short to properly activate the valves in the IV cassette. The result was a free flow condition. If the pump had been tested with the IV sets recommended for use with the pump, the recall probably could have been avoided.

likely to occur. These manufacturers should design and label their products to encourage proper use and to minimize the frequency of misuse.[15]

The design is typically approved after its technical adequacy has been verified through applicable testing. The design, which includes components, packaging and labeling, is then translated into approved, formal specifications. The device, however, is not yet ready to be released to manufacturing for routine production.

Before the specifications are released for routine production, actual finished devices should be manufactured using the approved specifications, the same materials and components, the same or similar production and quality control equipment, and the methods and procedures that will be used for routine production. Typically, this is accomplished by manufacturing "pilot runs" or "first production runs." These devices should then be qualified through extensive testing under actual or simulated use conditions and in the environment, or simulated environment, in which the device is expected to be used. The extent of the testing conducted should be governed by the risk the device will present should it fail. These procedures are considered essential for assuring the manufacturing process will produce the intended devices without adversely affecting the devices and are a necessary part of process validation.[16]

Caution should be taken when using prototypes developed in the laboratory or machine shop as qualification units. Prototypes may not be like the finished production device. During R&D, conditions are typically better controlled and personnel more knowledgeable about what needs to be done and how to do it than production personnel. When going from laboratory to scaled-up production, standards or methods and procedures may not be properly transferred or additional manufacturing processes may be added. Often changes, not reflected in the prototype, are made in the product to facilitate the manufacturing process. Proper qualification of devices that are produced using the same or similar methods and procedures as those to be used in routine

---

15. For example, an exhalation valve used in conjunction with a ventilator could be connected in a reverse position because the inlet and exhalation ports were the same diameter. In the reverse position the user could breath spontaneously but was isolated from the ventilator. The valve should have been designed so that it could be connected only in the proper position.

16. Food and Drug Administration, Center for Drugs and Biologics and Center for Devices and Radiological Health, "Guideline on General Principles of Process Validation," FDA, Rockville, Maryland, May 1987.

production can prevent the distribution and subsequent recall of many unacceptable medical devices.[17]

Typically, testing under use conditions is the clinical or in-vivo testing stage for devices requiring an Investigational Device Exemption (IDE), or clinical studies to support a Premarket Notification [510(k)], or Premarket Approval (PMA) submission to FDA. When practical, clinical testing should be conducted using devices produced under expected routine production conditions. Otherwise, the clinically qualified device will not be truly representative of production devices. Advice from clinicians should be sought with respect to how the device will actually be used. Testing should include stressing the device at its performance and environmental specification limits.[18]

Testing should be performed according to a documented test plan that specifies the performance parameters to be measured, test sequence, evaluation criteria, test environment, etc. Once the device is qualified, all manufacturing and quality assurance specifications should be placed under formal change control. Storage conditions should be considered when establishing environmental test specifications.[19, 20]

---

17. For example, a drainage catheter using a new material was designed, fabricated and subsequently qualified in a laboratory setting. Once the catheter was manufactured and distributed, however, the manufacturer began receiving complaints that the bifurcated sleeve was separating from the catheter shrink base. Investigation revealed the separation was a result of dimensional shrinkage of the material and leeching of the plasticizers from the sleeve due to exposure to cleaning solution during manufacturing. Had the device been exposed to actual production conditions during fabrication of the prototypes, the problem might have been detected before routine production and distribution.

18. For example, for an electrical device such as a cardiac monitor, electrical stress testing should include: device ON-OFF cycling, operation in accordance with all specified operating mode upper and lower limits and performance cycles, and input voltage variance above and below the nominal value. Such testing should be performed in the presence of electrical noise from such sources as electrical beds, electrocautery machines, and electrostatic discharge.

19. For example, a surgical staple device was recalled because it malfunctioned. Investigation showed that the device malfunctioned because of shrinkage of the plastic cutting ring resulting from the sub-zero conditions to which the device was exposed during shipping and storage.

20. In another example, a potassium electrode for use with a sodium/potassium analyzer was recalled because of complaints of low potassium level readings that were in error. Investigation determined that the solution that bathes the potassium electrode during shipping and storage was the cause of the erroneous readings.

3.9 Certification

After initial production units have successfully passed preproduction qualification testing, a formal technical review should be
conducted to assure adequacy of the design, production, and quality assurance procedures, and should include a determination of
the:

- Resolution of any differences between the procedures and
  standards used to produce the design while in R&D and
  those approved for production.

- Resolution of any differences between the approved device
  specifications and the actual manufactured product.

- Validity of test methods used to determine compliance
  with the approved specifications.

- Adequacy of specifications and specification change control program.

- Adequacy of the complete quality assurance plan.

3.10 Personnel

Design activities, including design review, analysis, and testing
should be conducted by appropriately trained and competent personnel.

3.11 Test Instrumentation

All equipment used in qualification of the design should be properly calibrated and maintained under a formal calibration and
maintenance program.

3.12 Quality Monitoring after the Design Phase

Once the design has been proven safe and effective and devices
are produced and distributed, the effort to assure that the device
and its components have acceptable quality and are safe and effective is not complete. This effort must be continued in the manufacturing and use phase.

Each medical device manufacturer must have an effective program for: identifying failure patterns or trends and analyzing quality problems; taking appropriate corrective action to prevent

recurrence of these problems; and timely internal reporting of problems discovered either in-house or in the field. Specific instructions should be established to provide direction about when and how problems are to be investigated, analyzed, and corrected, and to establish responsibility for assuring initiation and completion of these tasks.

When problem investigation and analysis indicate a potential problem in the design, appropriate design improvements must be made to prevent recurrence of the problem. Any design changes must undergo sufficient testing and preproduction evaluation to assure that the revised design is safe and effective. This testing should include testing under actual or simulated use conditions and clinical testing as appropriate to the change.

A special effort should be made to assure that failure data obtained from complaint and service records that may relate to design problems are made available and reviewed by those responsible for design.

Appendix A: Definitions

Certification	A documented review and approval of all qualification and validation documentation prior to release of the design for production.
Characteristic	A physical, chemical, visual, functional, or any other identifiable property of a medical device or part or material. (MIL-STD-109B)
Criticality	A relative measure of the consequences of a failure mode and its frequency of occurrence. (MIL-STD-1629A)
Defect	Any nonconformance of a characteristic with specified requirements. (MIL-STD-109B)
Design review	A planned, scheduled, and documented audit of all pertinent aspects of the design that can affect performance, safety or effectiveness.
Design specifications	A description of the physical and functional requirements for an article. In its initial form, the design specification is a statement of functional requirements with only general coverage of physical and test requirements.

The design specification evolves through the R&D phase to reflect progressive refinements in performance, design, configuration, and test requirements.

Design transfer

The transfer of the design basis or baseline into specifications for the device, its components, packaging, and labeling, and the manufacturing and quality assurance procedures, methods, specifications, etc., so that the device can be produced using production methods.

Environment

The conditions, circumstances, influences, and stresses surrounding and affecting the device during manufacture, storage, handling, transportation, installation, and use.

Failure

An event in which an article does not perform one or more of its required functions within the specified limits under specified conditions.

Failure analysis

The logical, systematic examination of an item, including its diagrams or formulas, to identify and analyze the probability, causes, and consequences of potential and real failures.

Failure effect

The consequences a failure has on the operation, function, or status of a device.

Failure mode

The manner in which a failure is observed. The way a failure occurs and its impact on the device performance (MIL-STD-109B).

Failure mode effects analysis

The process of identifying potential design weaknesses through reviewing schematics, engineering drawings, etc., to identify basic faults at the part/material level and to determine their effect at finished or subassembly level on safety and effectiveness (Reliability Design Handbook, RDG 376, Reliability Analysis Center, Rome Air Development Center).

Failure pattern	The occurrence of two or more failures of the same component or feature in identical or equivalent applications which are caused by the same basic failure mechanism. (MIL-STD-781C)
FDA recommendations	A means FDA uses to disseminate information tion about matters authorized by, but not involving direct regulatory action under, the laws the agency administers. Recommendations are not legally binding on manufacturers.
Nonconformance	A condition of any device or component in which one or more characteristics do not conform to requirements; includes failures, deficiencies, defects, and malfunctions.
Qualification	A documented determination that a device (and its associated software), component, packaging or labeling, meets all prescribed design and performance requirements.
Quality	The composite of all the characteristics, including performance, of an item or product (MIL-STD-109B)
Quality assurance	A planned and systematic pattern of all actions necessary to provide adequate confidence that the device, its components, packaging, and labeling are acceptable for their intended use.
Reliability	The characteristic of a device, or any component thereof, expressed as a probability that it will perform its required functions under defined conditions for specified operating periods.
Reliability assessment	A quantitative assessment of the reliability of a device, system, or portion thereof. Such assessments usually employ mathematical modeling, directly applicable results of tests on the device, failure data, estimated reliability figures, and nonstatistical

	engineering estimates (Reliability Design Handbook, RDG 376, Reliability Analysis Center, Rome Air Development Center).
Severity	The consequences of a failure mode. Severity considers the worst potential consequences of a failure, determined by the degree of injury.
System	The principal functioning entities comprising the device (for example, hardware and software). Also an organized and disciplined approach to accomplish a task (for example, a failure reporting system).
Testing	The determination by technical or scientific means of the properties or elements of a device or its components, including functional operation, and involving the application of established scientific principles and procedures.

Appendix B: References

Military Standards

1. MIL-STD-1629A   Procedures for Performing Failure Mode, Effects and Criticality Analysis

2. MIL-STD-785B   Reliability Program for Systems and Equipment Development and Production

3. MIL-STD-109B   Quality Assurance Terms and Definitions

4. MIL-STD-217B   Reliability Prediction of Electronic Equipment

5. MIL-STD-472   Maintainability Predictions

6. MIL-STD-1521A   Technical Reviews and Audits for Systems, Equipments, and Computer Programs

7. MIL-STD-781C   Reliability Design Qualification and Production Acceptance Tests: Exponential Distribution.

8. MIL-STD-483   Configuration Management

National Aeronautics and Space Administration

1. NASA SP-6502   Elements of Design Review for Space Systems

2. NASA SP-6504   Failure Reporting and Management Techniques in the Surveyor Program

3. NHB 5300.4(A)   Reliability Program Provisions for Aeronautical and Space System Contractors

4. N68-10120   Parts and Materials Application Review for Space Systems

5. N68-20357   An Introduction to the Assurance of Human Performance in Space Systems

Voluntary Standards

1. ANSI/ASQC Z-1.15-1979   Generic Guidelines for Quality Systems

2. ASQC C1-1968   Specification of General Requirements for a Quality Program

3. ANSI/IEEE STD 730-1984   IEEE Standard for Software Quality Assurance Plans

4. ANSI/IEEE STD 830-1981   Guide to Software Requirements Specifications

Appendix C: Quality Assurance Literature

1. Caplan, Frank, "The Quality System, A Source-book for Managers and Engineers." Chilton, Radnor, Pa. (1980).

2. Juran, J.M., "Quality Control Handbook." 3rd edition, McGraw-Hill, N.Y. (1974).

3. Lloyd, David K. & Lipow, Myron, "Reliability: Management, Methods, and Mathematics." Prentice-Hall, N.J. (1964).

Other

1. RDH-376 "Reliability Design Handbook." Reliability Analysis Center, Rome Air Development Center, Griffiss Air Force Base, N.Y. (1976).

2. NBS* Special Publication 500-98, "Planning for Software Validation, Verification, and Testing." (November 1982).

3. NBS* Special Publication 500-75, "Validation, Verification, and Testing of Computer Software." (February 1981).

4. NBS* Special Publication 500-56, "Validation, Verification, and Testing for the Individual Programmer." (February 1980).

NBS Federal Information Processing Standards Publications (FIPS PUBS)

1. FIPS PUB 38, "Guidelines for Documentation of Computer Programs and Automated Data Systems." (February 1976).

2. FIPS PUB 64, "Guidelines for Documentation of Computer Programs, and Automated Data Systems for the Initiation Phase." (August 1979).

3. FIPS PUB 101, "Guidelines for Lifecycle Validation, Verification, and Testing of Computer Software." (June 1983).

---

*NBS (National Bureau of Standards) is now the National Institute of Science and Technology.

Appendix C.2

Guideline on General Principles of Process Validation

Prepared by the Center for Drugs and Biologics and
the Center for Devices and Radiological Health
U.S. Food and Drug Administration
May, 1987

I.   Purpose

This guideline outlines general principles that FDA considers to be
acceptable elements of process validation for the preparation of
human and animal drug products and medical devices.

II.   Scope

This guideline is issued under Section 10.90 (21 CFR 10.90) and is
applicable to the manufacture of pharmaceuticals and medical devices. It states principles and practices of general applicability that
are not legal requirements but are acceptable to the FDA. A person
may rely upon this guideline with the assurance of its acceptability
to FDA, or may follow different procedures. When different procedures are used, a person may, but is not required to, discuss the

matter in advance with FDA to prevent the expenditure of money and effort on activities that may later be determined to be unacceptable. In short, this guideline lists principles and practices which are acceptable to the FDA for the process validation of drug products and medical devices; it does not list *the* principles and practices that must, in all instances, be used to comply with law.

This guideline may be amended from time to time. Interested persons are invited to submit comments on this document and any subsequent revisions. Written comments should be submitted to the Dockets Management Branch (HFA-305), Food and Drug Administration, Room 4-62, 5600 Fishers Lane, Rockville, Maryland 20857. Received comments may be seen in that office between 9 a.m. and 4 p.m., Monday through Friday.

III. Introduction

Process validation is a requirement of the Current Good Manufacturing Practices Regulations for Finished Pharmaceuticals, 21 CFR Parts 210 and 211, and of the Good Manufacturing Practice Regulations for Medical Devices, 21 CFR Part 820, and therefore, is applicable to the manufacture of pharmaceuticals and medical devices.

Several firms have asked FDA for specific guidance on what FDA expects firms to do to assure compliance with the requirements for process validation. This guideline discusses process validation elements and concepts that are considered by FDA as acceptable parts of a validation program. The constituents of validation presented in this document are not intended to be all-inclusive. FDA recognizes that, because of the great variety of medical products (drug products and medical devices), processes and manufacturing facilities, it is not possible to state in one document all of the specific validation elements that are applicable. Several broad concepts, however, have general applicability which manufacturers can use successfully as a guide in validating a manufacturing process. Although the particular requirements of process validation will vary according to such factors as the nature of the medical product (e.g., sterile vs non-sterile) and the complexity of the process, the broad concepts stated in this document have general applicability and provide an acceptable framework for building a comprehensive approach to process validation.

Definitions

Installation qualification—Establishing confidence that process equipment and ancillary systems are capable of consistently operating within established limits and tolerances.

Process performance qualification—Establishing confidence that the process is effective and reproducible.

Product performance qualification—Establishing confidence through appropriate testing that the finished product produced by a specified process meets all release requirements for functionality and safety.

Prospective validation—Validation conducted prior to the distribution of either a new product, or product made under a revised manufacturing process, where the revisions may affect the product's characteristics.

Retrospective validation—Validation of a process for a product already in distribution based upon accumulated production, testing and control data.

Validation—Establishing documented evidence which provides a high degree of assurance that a specific process will consistently produce a product meeting its pre-determined specifications and quality attributes.

Validation protocol—A written plan stating how validation will be conducted, including test parameters, product characteristics, production equipment, and decision points on what constitutes acceptable test results.

Worst case—A set of conditions encompassing upper and lower processing limits and circumstances, including those within standard operating procedures, which pose the greatest chance of process or product failure when compared to ideal conditions. Such conditions do not necessarily induce product or process failure.

IV.   General Concepts

Assurance of product quality is derived from careful attention to a number of factors including selection of quality parts and materials, adequate product and process design, control of the process, and in-process and end-product testing. Due to the complexity of today's medical products, routine end-product testing alone often is not sufficient to assure product quality for several reasons. Some end-product tests have limited sensitivity.[1] In some cases, destructive testing would be required to show that the manufacturing process was adequate, and in other situations end-product testing does not reveal all variations that may occur in the product that may impact on safety and effectiveness.[2]

The basic principles of quality assurance have as their goal the production of articles that are fit for their intended use. These principles may be stated as follows: (1) quality, safety, and effectiveness must be designed and built into the product; (2) quality cannot be inspected or tested into the finished product; and (3) each step of the manufacturing process must be controlled to maximize the probability that the finished product meets all quality and design specifications. Process validation is a key element in assuring that these quality assurance goals are met.

It is through careful design and validation of both the process and process controls that a manufacturer can establish a high degree of confidence that all manufactured units from successive lots will be acceptable. Successfully validating a process may reduce the dependence upon intensive in-process and finished product testing. It should be noted that in most all cases, end-product testing plays a major role in assuring that quality assurance goals are met; i.e., validation and end-product testing are not mutually exclusive.

The FDA defines process validation as follows:

Process validation is establishing documented evidence which provides a high degree of assurance that a specific process will consistently produce a product meeting its pre-determined specifications and quality characteristics.

It is important that the manufacturer prepare a written validation protocol which specifies the procedures (and tests) to be conducted and the data to be collected. The purpose for which data

---

1   For example, USP XXI states: "No sampling plan for applying sterility tests to a specified proportion of discrete units selected from a sterilization load is capable of demonstrating with complete assurance that all of the untested units are in fact sterile."

2   As an example, in one instance a visual inspection failed to detect a defective structural weld which resulted in the failure of an infant warmer. The defect could only have been detected by using destructive testing or expensive test equipment.

are collected must be clear, the data must reflect facts and be collected carefully and accurately. The protocol should specify a sufficient number of replicate process runs to demonstrate reproducibility and provide an accurate measure of variability among successive runs. The test conditions for these runs should encompass upper and lower processing limits and circumstances, including those within standard operating procedures, which pose the greatest chance of process or product failure compared to ideal conditions; such conditions have become widely known as "worst case" conditions. (They are sometimes called "most appropriate challenge" conditions.) Validation documentation should include evidence of the suitability of materials and the performance and reliability of equipment and systems.

Key process variables should be monitored and documented. Analysis of the data collected from monitoring will establish the variability of process parameters for individual runs and will establish whether or not the equipment and process controls are adequate to assure that product specifications are met.

Finished product and in-process test data can be of value in process validation, particularly in those situations where quality attributes and variabilities can be readily measured. Where finished (or in-process) testing cannot adequately measure certain attributes, process validation should be derived primarily from qualification of each system used in production and from consideration of the interaction of the various systems.

V. CGMP Regulations for Finished Pharmaceuticals

Process validation is required, in both general and specific terms, by the Current Good Manufacturing Practice Regulations for Finished Pharmaceuticals, 21 CFR Parts 210 and 211. Examples of such requirements are listed below for informational purposes, and are not all-inclusive.

A requirement for process validation is set forth in general terms in section 211.100—Written procedures; deviations—which states, in part:

"There shall be written procedures for production and process control designed to assure that the drug products have the identity, strength, quality, and purity they purport or are represented to possess."

Several sections of the CGMP regulations state validation requirements in more specific terms. Excerpts from some of these sections are:

Section 211.110, Sampling and testing of in-process materials and drug products.

(a) " . . . . control procedures shall be established to monitor the output and VALIDATE the performance of those manufacturing processes that may be responsible for causing variability in the characteristics of in-process material and the drug product." (emphasis added)

Section 211.113, Control of Microbiological Contamination.

(b) "Appropriate written procedures, designed to prevent microbiological contamination of drug products purporting to be sterile, shall be established and followed. Such procedures shall include VALIDATION of any sterilization process." (emphasis added)

VI.   GMP Regulation for Medical Devices

Process validation is required by the medical device GMP Regulations, 21 CFR Part 820. Section 820.5 requires every finished device manufacturer to:

" . . . prepare and implement a quality assurance program that is appropriate to the specific device manufactured . . . "

Section 820.3(n) defines quality assurance as:

" . . . all activities necessary to verify confidence in the quality of the process used to manufacture a finished device."

When applicable to a specific process, process validation is an essential element in establishing confidence that a process will consistently produce a product meeting the designed quality characteristics.

A generally stated requirement for process validation is contained in section 820.100:

"Written manufacturing specifications and processing procedures shall be established, implemented, and controlled to assure that the device conforms to its original design or any approved changes in that design."

Validation is an essential element in the establishment and implementation of a process procedure, as well as in determining what process controls are required in order to assure conformance to specifications.

Section 820.100(a)(1) states:

" . . . control measures shall be established to assure that the design basis for the device, components and packaging is correctly translated into approved specifications."

Validation is an essential control for assuring that the specifications for the device and manufacturing process are adequate to produce a device that will conform to the approved design characteristics.

VII.   Preliminary Considerations

A manufacturer should evaluate all factors that affect product quality when designing and undertaking a process validation study. These factors may vary considerably among different products and manufacturing technologies and could include, for example, component specifications, air and water handling systems, environmental controls, equipment functions, and process control operations. No single approach to process validation will be appropriate and complete in all cases; however, the following quality activities should be undertaken in most situations.

During the research and development (R&D) phase, the desired product should be carefully defined in terms of its characteristics, such as physical, chemical, electrical and performance characteristics.[3] It is important to translate the product character-

---

3   For example, in the case of a compressed tablet, physical characteristics would include size, weight, hardness, and freedom from defects, such as capping and splitting. Chemical characteristics would include quantitative formulation/potency; performance characteristics may include bioavailability (reflected by disintegration ad dissolution). In the case of blood tubing, physical attributes would include internal and external diameters, length and color. Chemical characteristics would include raw material formulation. Mechanical properties would include hardness and tensile strength; performance characteristics would include biocompatibility and durability.

istics into specifications as a basis for description and control of the product.

Documentation of changes made during development provide traceability which can later be used to pinpoint solutions to future problems.

The product's end use should be a determining factor in the development of product (and component) characteristics and specifications. All pertinent aspects of the product which impact on safety and effectiveness should be considered. These aspects include performance, reliability and stability. Acceptable ranges or limits should be established for each characteristic to set up allowable variations.[4] These ranges should be expressed in readily measurable terms.

The validity of acceptance specifications should be verified through testing and challenge of the product on a sound scientific basis during the initial development and production phase.

Once a specification is demonstrated as acceptable it is important that any changes to the specification be made in accordance with documented change control procedures.

VIII. Elements of Process Validation

A. Prospective Validation

Prospective validation includes those considerations that should be made before an entirely new product is introduced by a firm or when there is a change in the manufacturing process which may affect the product's characteristics, such as uniformity and identity. The following are considered as key elements of prospective validation.

1. Equipment and Process

The equipment and process(es) should be designed and/or selected so that product specifications are consistently achieved. This should be done with the participation of all appropriate groups that are concerned with assuring a quality product, e.g., engineering design, production operations, and quality assurance personnel.

---

4   For example, in order to assure that an oral, ophthalmic, or parenteral solution has an acceptable pH, a specification may be established by which a lot is released only if it has been shown to have a pH within a narrow established range. For a device, a specification for the electrical resistance of a pacemaker lead would be established so that the lead would be acceptable only if the resistance was within a specified range.

a. Equipment: Installation Qualification

Installation qualification studies establish confidence that the process equipment and ancillary systems are capable of consistently operating within established limits and tolerances. After process equipment is designed or selected, it should be evaluated and tested to verify that it is capable of operating satisfactorily within the operating limits required by the process.[5] This phase of validation includes examination of equipment design; determination of calibration, maintenance, and adjustment requirements; and identifying critical equipment features that could affect the process and product. Information obtained from these studies should be used to establish written procedures covering equipment calibration, maintenance, monitoring, and control.

In assessing the suitability of a given piece of equipment, it is usually insufficient to rely solely upon the representations of the equipment supplier, or upon experience in producing some other product.[6] Sound theoretical and practical engineering principles and considerations are a first step in the assessment.

It is important that equipment qualification simulate actual production conditions, including those which are "worst case" situations.

Tests and challenges should be repeated a sufficient number of times to assure reliable and meaningful results. All acceptance

---

5 Examples of equipment performance characteristics which may be measured include temperature and pressure of injection molding machines, uniformity of speed for mixers, temperature, speed and pressure for packaging machines, and temperature and pressure of sterilization chambers.

6 The importance of assessing equipment suitability based upon how it will be used to attain desired product attributes is illustrated in the case of deionizers used to produce Purified Water, USP. In one case, a firm used such water to make a topical drug product solution which, in view of its intended use, should have been free from objectionable microorganisms. However, the product was found to be contaminated with a pathogenic microorganism. The apparent cause of the problem was failure to assess the performance of the deionizer from a microbiological standpoint. It is fairly well recognized that the deionizers are prone to build-up of microorganisms—especially if the flow rates are low and the deionizers are not recharged and sanitized at suitable intervals. Therefore, these factors should have been considered. In this case, however, the firm relied upon the representations of the equipment itself, namely the "recharge" (i.e., conductivity) indicator, to signal the time for regeneration and cleaning. Considering the desired product characteristics, the firm should have determined the need for such procedures based upon pre-use testing, taking into account such factors as the length of time the equipment could produce deionized water of acceptable quality, flow rate, temperature, raw water quality, frequency of use, and surface area of deionizing resins.

criteria must be met during the test or challenge. If any test or challenge shows that the equipment does not perform within its specifications, an evaluation should be performed to identify the cause of the failure. Corrections should be made and additional test runs performed, as needed, to verify that the equipment performs within specifications. The observed variability of the equipment between and within runs can be used as a basis for determining the total number of trials selected for the subsequent performance qualification studies of the process.[7]

Once the equipment configuration and performance characteristics are established and qualified, they should be documented. The installation qualification should include a review of pertinent maintenance procedures, repair parts lists, and calibration methods for each piece of equipment. The objective is to assure that all repairs can be performed in such a way that will not affect the characteristics of material processed after the repair. In addition, special post-repair cleaning and calibration requirements should be developed to prevent inadvertent manufacture of a non-conforming product. Planning during the qualification phase can prevent confusion during emergency repairs which could lead to use of the wrong replacement part.

b. Process: Performance Qualification

The purpose of performance qualification is to provide rigorous testing to demonstrate the effectiveness and reproducibility of the process. In entering the performance qualification phase of validation, it is understood that the process specifications have been established and essentially proven acceptable through laboratory or other trial methods and that the equipment has been judged acceptable on the basis of suitable installation studies.

Each process should be defined and described with sufficient specificity so that employees understand what is required.

Parts of the process which may vary so as to affect important product quality should be challenged.[8]

---

7   For example, the AAMI Guideline for Industrial Ethylene Oxide Sterilization of Medical Devices approved 2 December 1981, states: "The performance qualification should include a minimum of 3 successful, planned qualification runs, in which all of the acceptance criteria are met . . . . . " (5.3.1.2.).

8   For example, in electroplating the metal case of an implantable pacemaker, the significant process steps to define, describe, and challenge include establishment and control of current density and temperature values for assuring adequate composition of electrolyte and for assuring cleanliness of the metal to

In challenging a process to assess its adequacy, it is important that challenge conditions simulate those that will be encountered during actual production, including "worst case" conditions. The challenges should be repeated enough times to assure that the results are meaningful and consistent.

Each specific manufacturing process should be appropriately qualified and validated. There is an inherent danger in relying on what are perceived to be similarities between products, processes, and equipment without appropriate challenge.[9]

c. Product: Performance Qualification

For purposes of this guideline, product performance qualification activities apply only to medical devices. These steps should be viewed as pre-production quality assurance activities.

Before reaching the conclusion that a process has been successfully validated, it is necessary to demonstrate that the specified process has not adversely affected the finished product. Where possible, product performance qualification testing should include performance testing under conditions that simulate actual use. Product performance qualification testing should be conducted using product manufactured from the same type of production equipment, methods and procedures that will be used for routine production. Otherwise, the qualified product may not be representative of production units and cannot be used as evidence

---

8   *continued*
   be plated. In the production of parenteral solutions by aseptic filling, the significant aseptic filling process steps to define and challenge should include the sterilization and depyrogenation of containers/closures, sterilization of solutions, filling equipment and product contact surfaces, and the filling and closing of containers.

9   For example, in the production of a compressed tablet, a firm may switch from one type of granulation blender to another with the erroneous assumption that both types have similar performance characteristics, and, therefore, granulation mixing times and procedures need not be altered. However, if the blenders are substantially different, use of the new blender with procedures used for the previous blender may result in a granulation with poor content uniformity. This, in turn, may lead to tablets having significantly differing potencies. This situation may be averted if the quality assurance system detects the equipment change in the first place, challenges the blender performance, precipitates a revalidation of the process, and initiates appropriate changes. In this example, revalidation comprises installation qualification of the new equipment and performance qualification of the process intended for use in the new blender.

that the manufacturing process will produce a product that meets the pre-determined specifications and quality attributes.[10]

After actual production units have successfully passed product performance qualification, a formal technical review should be conducted and should include:

- Comparison of the approved product specifications and the actual qualified product.

- Determination of the validity of test methods used to determine compliance with the approved specifications.

- Determination of the adequacy of the specification change control program.

2.   System to Assure Timely Revalidation

There should be a quality assurance system in place which requires revalidation whenever there are changes in packaging, formulation, equipment, or processes which could impact on product effectiveness or product characteristics, and whenever there are changes in product characteristics. Furthermore, when a change is made in raw material supplier, the manufacturer should consider subtle, potentially adverse differences in the raw material characteristics. A determination of adverse differences in raw material indicates a need to revalidate the process.

One way of detecting the kind of changes that should initiate revalidation is the use of tests and methods of analysis which are capable of measuring characteristics which may vary. Such tests

---

10   For example, a manufacturer of heart valves received complaints that the valve-support structure was fracturing under use. Investigation by the manufacturer revealed that all material and dimensional specifications had been met but the production machining process created microscopic scratches on the valve supporting wireform. These scratches caused metal fatigue and subsequent fracture. Comprehensive fatigue testing of production units under simulated use conditions could have detected the process deficiency.

In another example, a manufacturer recalled insulin syringes because of complaints that the needles were clogged. Investigation revealed that the needles were clogged by silicone oil which was employed as a lubricant during manufacturing. Investigation further revealed that the method used to extract the silicone oil was only partially effective. Although visual inspection of the syringes seemed to support that the cleaning method was effective, actual use proved otherwise.

and methods usually yield specific results which go beyond the mere pass/fail basis, thereby detecting variations within product and process specifications and allowing determination of whether a process is slipping out of control.

The quality assurance procedures should establish the circumstances under which revalidation is required. These may be based upon equipment, process, and product performance observed during the initial validation challenge studies. It is desirable to designate individuals who have the responsibility to review product, process, equipment and personnel changes to determine if and when revalidation is warranted.

The extent of revalidation will depend upon the nature of the changes and how they impact upon different aspects of production that had previously been validated. It may not be necessary to revalidate a process from scratch merely because a given circumstance has changed. However, it is important to carefully assess the nature of the change to determine potential ripple effects and what needs to be considered as part of revalidation.

3. Documentation

It is essential that the validation program is documented and that the documentation is properly maintained. Approval and release of the process for use in routine manufacturing should be based upon a review of all the validation documentation, including data from the equipment qualification, process performance qualification, and product/package testing to ensure compatibility with the process.

For routine production, it is important to adequately record process details (e.g., time, temperature, equipment used) and to record any changes which have occurred. A maintenance log can be useful in performing failure investigations concerning a specific manufacturing lot. Validation data (along with specific test data) may also determine expected variance in product or equipment characteristics.

B. Retrospective Process Validation

In some cases a product may have been on the market without sufficient premarket process validation. In these cases, it may be possible to validate, in some measure, the adequacy of the process by examination of accumulated test data on the product and records of the manufacturing procedures used.

Retrospective validation can also be useful to augment initial premarket prospective validation for new products or changed processes. In such cases, preliminary prospective validation should have been sufficient to warrant product marketing. As additional data is gathered on production lots, such data can be used to build confidence in the adequacy of the process. Conversely, such data may indicate a declining confidence in the process and a commensurate need for corrective changes.

Test data may be useful only if the methods and results are adequately specific. As with prospective validation, it may be insufficient to assess the process solely on the basis of lot by lot conformance to specifications if test results are merely expressed in terms of pass/fail. Specific results, on the other hand, can be statistically analyzed and a determination can be made of what variance in data can be expected. It is important to maintain records which describe the operating characteristics of the process, e.g., time, temperature, humidity, and equipment settings.[11] Whenever test data are used to demonstrate conformance to specifications, it is important that the test methodology be qualified to assure that test results are objective and accurate.

IX.   Acceptability of Product Testing

In some cases, a drug product or medical device may be manufactured individually or on a one-time basis. The concept of prospective or retrospective validation as it relates to those situations may have limited applicability, and data obtained during the manufacturing and assembly process may be used in conjunction with product testing to demonstrate that the instant run yielded a finished product meeting all of its specifications and quality characteristics. Such evaluation of data and product testing would be expected to be much more extensive than the usual situation where more reliance would be placed on prospective validation.

---

11 For example, sterilizer time and temperature data collected on recording equipment found to be accurate and precise could establish that process parameters had been reliably delivered to previously processed loads. A retrospective qualification of the equipment could be performed to demonstrate that the recorded data represented conditions that were uniform throughout the chamber and that product load configurations, personnel practices, initial temperature, and other variables had been adequately controlled during the earlier runs.

Appendix C.3

Contract Sterilization Guidelines (Draft)

Introduction

Written agreements between medical device manufacturers and contract sterilizers are needed to assure compliance with regulatory, technical and business requirements. This section will delineate the regulations, technical parameters, and control activities related to these agreements.

It is common industry practice for a manufacturer to produce and/or assemble, package and fully label devices as sterile at one establishment and then ship the devices to a contract sterilizer for sterilization and return to the manufacturer or other consignee. Throughout this complete series of events, the manufacturer and contract sterilizer must meet the applicable requirements in 21 CFR Section 801.150, "Medical devices; processing, labeling, or repacking" and 21 CFR Part 820, "Manufacture, Packing, Storage, and Installation of Medical Devices" (GMPs). Also, Section 801.150 requires that a written agreement be obtained between the person shipping the non-sterile device and the operator or person in charge of the establishment receiving the device for sterilization. Part 820 requires that all processing be done under GMP conditions.

Contract sterilization is an extension of the finished device manufacturer's process (820.3(k)). The device manufacturer is ultimately responsible for assuring that all manufacturing and sterilization operations plus quality assurance checks used for the devices are appropriate, adequate, and correctly performed (820.5).

Contract sterilizers, however, are responsible for and are subject to regulatory inspections for those sections of the GMP that apply to the manufacturing operation they perform for finished device manufacturers—e.g., equipment maintenance and calibration, in-process controls, and associated recordkeeping.

Since the manufacturer has the primary responsibility for the sterility of his device, he must do more than execute a business-only agreement with the contract sterilizer. The manufacturer must see that each party plans, agrees on, executes and controls an overall documented process that will assure sterile devices and compliance with the medical device regulations.

Scope of the Agreement

The agreement should cover the device(s) to be sterilized and cover the required actions of the contract sterilizer, actions of the manufacturer and mutual activities. The activities include:

validation	records
bioburden control	approvals
labeling	documentation control
secondary packaging	process control
receipt and handling	information transfer and
preconditioning	contacts
biological indicators	non-conformance
loading	reprocessing
cycle parameters	maintenance
cycle control & records	calibration
post handling	training
shipping	audits

Some of these activities will be discussed briefly in the remainder of this guideline with emphasis on the responsibility of each party. This guideline does not cover the multitude of related business factors such as:

costs/prices/charges	length of agreement
product insurance	extent of agreement
extended storage of product	indemnification clauses

termination of agreement
what takes precedence

Federal, State, and Local Laws
acts of nature

Where various devices that require different sterilization cycles are to be processed by a contract sterilizer, a general agreement may be used to cover the GMP and other non-device specific items; and a supplemental agreement can be used to cover the device-specific items such as cycle parameters or special handling. The general agreement may refer to specifications on the manufacturer's purchase order that become binding when the purchase order is accepted and acknowledged by the contract sterilizer.

Device Process Compatibility

At the beginning of the agreement negotiations, the manufacturer may wish to list the device and primary package characteristics, outline his GMP system for bioburden control (820.25, 820.40, 820.46, 820.56, 820.60, 820.130), note any desired sterilization parameters, and emphasize the need for GMP controls by both parties. The contract sterilizer may wish to respond with an overview of his GMP system and the characteristics of the sterilization process. Of course, the device and sterilization process must be compatible or capable of being made compatible in order to proceed with the agreement.

Training

It is necessary that the manufacturer assure himself that the entire sterilization process is performed and controlled by properly trained operators (820.25). The training should be documented and the agreement should state that the manufacturer will have access to training records during agreed-upon audits.

Information Transfer and Contacts

The manufacturer and contract sterilizer should designate individuals at each facility to send, receive, file and distribute important technical and device flow information. If a purchase order contains any part of the technical parameters which requires acknowledgement, it should pass through these designers as part of the routing.

There should be a timely flow of all applicable information between the parties. The information includes device flow, technical parameters, history records, problems and changes. Section 801.150(e) and the GMPs (part 820) require the important aspects of this information to be documented. Records should be made of applicable meetings, assignments and actions.

Documentation Change Control

The parties should certify that their applicable device process and control information is documented and controlled according to the requirements of the GMP (820.181). It is recommended that the parties be specific in reviewing and understanding their documentation control systems since both parties may have to generate, transfer, understand and execute interrelated documentation and changes in a timely and controlled manner. For documentation additions or changes, the parties must each have a self-approved procedure that is followed from the time a document is added or changed to the ultimate completion of the change. The two procedures should include the following activities:

> Identification of the change;
> Examination of the change related to the entire manufacturing process;
> Proof that the change achieves the desired results;
> Approvals;
> Document number and revision level;
> Effectivity date or action message;
> Disposition of in-process devices and components;
> Primary and secondary documentation updating;
> Distribution of the changed documentation (acknowledgement may be important in some cases);
> Obsolete document disposition;
> Coherence of the Master Record, History Record, History Record Forms and the first devices after the change.

The parties can select from the documentation control system any specific items that need to be referenced in the agreement. Particular attention should be paid to mutual items such as document distribution, disposition of in-process devices and control of obsolete documents.

Both parties must have designated individuals for approving the history records, the release of product, and any other agreed upon factor (820.150, 820.160, 820.161, 820.184, 820.185).

Approvals

Both parties must have designated individuals for approving the history records, the release of products, and any other agreed upon factor (820.150, 820.160, 820.161, 820.184, 820.185).

GMP Audits

Since contract sterilization is an extension of the device manufacturer's production process, GMP audits of the contractor must be performed by or reviewed by the manufacturer and corrective actions taken by the appropriate parties. The agreement should cover the extent of the audit, the frequency, corrective actions, records, confidentiality and the auditor (820.20).

Non-Conformance and Corrective Action

The parties must mutually inform each other if the device or process deviates from the agreed upon specifications. The parties must inform each other if the finished devices are found to be non-sterile or degraded or if the primary package is compromised. As appropriate, (See 820.162, 820.198, 820.20(a)(3)) the non-conformance must be investigated by the parties and corrective actions instituted.

The agreement should specify the procedure to be followed by the contractor when a device deficiency is noted, the sterilization equipment malfunctions or the process fails to meet the process specifications including testing and release criteria. Because of device storage factors, the manufacturer must respond to the contractor's disposition requests in a timely manner (for example, 24 hours).

The parties must consider, agree on and document the conditions for reprocessing (820.115, 820.116). The additional degradation and chemical residues due to reprocessing must be determined during qualification if reprocessing is to be allowed.

Qualification of Sterilization Process (Validation)

The manufacturer should work with the contract sterilizer to qualify the facilities, instrumentation and process in order to produce sterile devices (820.1, 820.100, 501(c), 502(a)). Records must be maintained of the qualification process. The agreement should specify all parameters to be qualified by the contractor and the criteria and the frequency which requalification will be required.

Cycle specifications should be clearly written for qualified cycles which define in detail the process parameters for each specific manufacturer's device or device family. The sample agreement at the end of this article contains a form for listing the sterilization cycle and product handling parameters. The agreement should define the records to be maintained of the measurements taken for each lot of devices to be sterilized per these specifications.

Product Load Configuration

The agreement should specify the loading parameters for each device or device family to be sterilized in lots (820.100, 820.101). The parameters to be specified include:

- Specifications of dissimilar devices which can be combined and those which cannot be combined in one sterilization load and identical cycle.

- Sequence of transfer of pallets to the sterilizer

- Physical separation of containers and pallets in the sterilizer both horizontally and vertically.

- Specific pallet diagram or pattern with top and side view. (The diagram must be approved, signed and change controlled.)

- Minimum and maximum number of units per pallet and per chamber when chambers can be specified.

- Agreement on handling of partial loads or shared loads.

- Location of Biological Indicators or inoculated samples.

Process Control

Once the overall sterilization process is qualified, it is essential that the contractor maintain control over the system to ensure that process specifications are routinely achieved (820.20). Since the contractor may perform sterilization services for many manufacturers and dissimilar devices, it is essential that each cycle qualified for a specific device and manufacturer be carefully documented, installed and monitored (820.100, 820.60(d), 820.181). This variation of cycle designs for various clients introduces additional quality control variables that must be considered and monitored by the manufacturer in evaluating the quality of services received from the contractor.

Process control includes verifying that the bio-indicators (spore strips), dosimeters, ethylene oxide and any other materials used in the overall sterilization process meet specifications. The verification is done by internal testing or by vendor as shown by the accompanying certificate of compliance. There certificate should list the key data.

Bio-Indicators and Test Samples

The agreement must define placement and/or recovery and handling by the contractor of product samples and any biological or chemical indicators (820.160, 820.161). The definition should include:

- Exactly where within primary or secondary packaging the indicators will be placed.

- Clear definition of markings on packages with bio-indicators which have been prepared by the manufacturer rather than the contract sterilizer.

- Instructions to the contractor for the removal, handling, and disposition of post-sterilized devices with included bio-indicators and the removal and disposition of control devices from the same carton.

- Instructions for replacing samples and/or marking cartons from which samples have been removed.

- Instruction on bio-indicator and post-sterilization sampling specifications to be followed by contractor.

- Instruction to contractor for packaging and shipment of bio-indicator and product samples to a testing laboratory for analysis.

- Instruction for shipment and/or storage of post-sterilized devices before and after release (820.150).

Process Change Control

The manufacturer as well as the contract sterilizer must agree to inform one another of any changes that may require re-qualification of the cycles. Examples of such changes include: variations in bioburden on raw materials or pre-sterilized product; packaging, device design, material or component changes; product defects or performance deficiencies; cycle failures or aberrations; control system bio-indicator or metrology problems; sterilizer modifications; and manufacturer or contractor environment or facility changes. The agreement should contain the procedure for mutual notification of these changes. Intentional changes that impact both parties should be approved by the manufacturer and the contractor.

Handling and Documentation

Product should be handled in a manner that prevents adulteration and damage and that absolutely segregates pre-sterilization and post-sterilization products under all foreseeable circumstances (See 801.150, 820.120, 820.150). Also, the manufacturer defines the "designated shipping unit" to be labeled. This may be a carton, a pallet or a full truck load. The following outline summarizes a general process for material handling and specifies the party that is usually responsible for each step.

1.0 Shipping from Manufacturer (Responsibility: Manufacturer)

1.1   Package the units to maintain product and primary package integrity and cleanliness.

1.2   Obtain signed agreement prior to first shipment.

1.3   Accurately determine and record number of units and test units shipped.

1.4 Conspicuously mark each pallet, carton, or other designated unit to show its non-sterile nature, e.g., NON-STERILE; SHIPPED FOR FURTHER PROCESSING.

1.5 Identify the product and the sterilization process specification to be used.

2.0 Receiving at the Contract Sterilizer (Responsibility: Contractor)

2.1 The product is identified versus the accompanying documents and agreed upon processing specifications.

2.2 The number of units received should be accurately determined and recorded; discrepancies are resolved with shipper.

2.3 Material is segregated by defined means in order to preclude accidental mixing with sterilized products.

2.4 Damaged material is documented and handled in the agreed upon manner.

2.5 Devices are stored in the agreed preconditioning environments.

3.0 Sterilization (Responsibility: Contractor)

3.1 The sterilizer is properly cleaned and the agreed upon cycle parameters are set.

3.2 The number of units going into the sterilizer is accurately determined and recorded.

3.3 The number of units coming out of the sterilizer is accurately determined and recorded.

3.4 The flow of material to and from the sterilization area is designed to prevent mixing of sterilized and unsterilized devices.

3.5 Sterilization cycle parameters that actually occurred during the processing are documented, signed by an operator, reviewed and approved/released by a supervisor.

4.0 Shipment from a Contractor (Responsibility: Contractor)

4.1 Test Devices Sent to Test Facilities

    a. The number of units shipped is accurately determined and recorded.

        b.   Each designated shipping unit is conspicuously marked, STERILIZED—TEST MATERIAL ONLY.

4.2   Processed Devices Returned to Manufacturer

        a.   The number of units shipped is accurately determined and recorded; differences should be resolved.

        b.   Each designated shipping unit is conspicuously marked, "STERILIZED—AWAITING TEST RESULTS."

        c.   If a Manufacturer's release is obtained, the devices may be shipped without over labeling.

5.0 Receiving at the Manufacturer (Responsibilities: Manufacturer)

5.1   Accurately determine and record number of units received. Discrepancies with the shipper should be resolved.

5.2   The processing records are reviewed by a designated individual and signed.

6.0 Receiving at the Test Facility (Responsibility: Test Facility and Manufacturer)

6.1   Accurately determine and record the number of test units received; discrepancies with the shipper should be resolved.

Outline of Sample Agreement for Contract Sterilization

This agreement* between the Manufacturer and the Contract Sterilizer (or Contractor) (insert names and addresses of the firms) covers the respective good manufacturing practices (GMPs) of both parties relative to medical devices produced or supplied by the manufacturer and the sterilization of the same devices by the Contractor.

Supplemental Agreement: The detailed sterilization cycle parameters and design parameters related to sterilization for the specific medical device are covered by a supplemental agreement attached hereto, and incorporated herein. The supplemental agreement may be a purchase order that contains the required parameters. The purchase order becomes binding when accepted and acknowledged by the Contractor.

Information Transfer and Contacts

The Manufacturer designates the employee with the position title of _____ and the Contractor designates the employee with the position title of _____ at their respective facilities to be responsible for the sending, receiving, filing and distribution of technical and product flow information.

---

* The actual agreement must be written to meet the Manufacturer's and Contractor's legal and GMP requirements. Likewise, the actual supplemental agreement must be written to meet specific device and process requirements. Some factors not listed in this outline are:

Cost/price changes	length of the agreement
product insurance	extent of the agreement
extended storage	indemnification
termination of the agreement	Federal, State, and Local Laws
what takes precedence	acts of nature
best effort re confidentiality	

(Note: This educational material is not an official statement binding FDA.)

Documentation

For the specific devices and processes covered by this supplemental agreement, or by acknowledged purchase orders, the parties agree to use only approved and signed documentation or record forms for devices to be released as sterile into commercial distribution.

For released documentation that has been exchanged, the parties agree to consult on proposed subsequent changes that could affect the sterility of the device and to exchange approved changed documentation in a timely manner.

GMPs and GMP Audit

For any appropriate good manufacturing practice not delineated in this agreement or the supplemental agreement, the parties agree to comply with the GMP regulation, (21 CFR 820) for the specific product and process identified in each supplemental agreement.

The Contractor agrees to use only appropriately trained operators for each aspect of the relevant processes and agrees to maintain records of future training.

The Contractor agrees to maintain and calibrate all relevant equipment in accordance with the Contractor's documented schedules and procedures and agrees to maintain records of the maintenance and calibration.

The parties agree to perform self-audits at least once a year and correct any relevant deficiency in the quality assurance system that covers the specific device and process identified in any current agreement or supplemental agreement and to inform each other when the audit is performed. Upon request to the Contractor, the Manufacturer shall be supplied a copy of the sections of the Contractor's audit report that are relevant to the processing covered by the agreement.

Representatives of the manufacturer shall be allowed access to the premises of the Contractor during ordinary business hours of the Contractor for inspecting or auditing the processing of the devices covered herein, for inspecting or auditing relevant maintenance, calibration, processing and training records and for

---

Validation

The parties agree to use a validated cycle for the sterilization of each device or compatible family of devices.

The parties agree to cooperate in validating and documenting the sterilization process.

The Contractor agrees to assign a control number to each documented, approved and validated sterilization cycle (See Documentation). Subsequent to validation, the parties agree to revalidate if the device fails to meet the agreed upon sterility specification and no other cause for failure can be determined after diligent investigation by the parties in their respective areas.

Sterilization Process Parameters

The detailed sterilization parameters established and validated for each device or family of devices are listed or referenced by a Specific Device Supplemental Agreement for Contract Sterilization attached hereto and incorporated herein. The supplemental agreement also covers specific handling, specific history records and device disposition.

Product and Process Change Control

After validation, the parties agree to inform each other, prior to the actual change, of any planned change in the components, device design, processing, packaging, handling, bioburden control, sterilization process or other factor known to have a significant bearing on the sterility of the finished device.

See Non-Conformance and also Documentation.

Bioburden Control

The Manufacturer certifies that the devices are processed under a documented bioburden control program. If requested by the Contractor, the Manufacturer agrees to supply a copy or summary of the bioburden history record(s) with each shipment (or other appropriate quantity) of devices to the Contractor.

Release Approvals

The Manufacturer agrees to release to the Contractor only devices that have been released by the designated authority of the Manufacturer and which meet the design and manufacturing specifications related to sterilization. The process records shall be signed by the designee to verify the review, compliance and release.

The Contractor agrees to release to the Manufacturer only devices that have been released by the Contractor's designated authority as having been processed according to this agreement, and the supplemental agreement for the specific device. The process records shall be signed by the designee to verify the review, compliance and release.

Shipping and Handling

For each shipment to the Contractor, the Manufacturer agrees to state on the accompanying documents his facility address, signature of the release authority, the device, the supplemental agreement number or sterilization specification number, the number of units, the date, and the lot or control numbers.

The Manufacturer agrees to mark the shipment of devices such that the supplemental agreement or purchase order can be readily identified that, in turn, identifies the cycle parameters to be used by the Contractor to sterilize the specific device.

The Manufacturer agrees to mark each pallet, carton, or other designated unit to show its nonsterile nature.

Following sterilization, and until such time as it is established that the device is sterile and can be released from quarantine, the Contractor agrees to show that it has not been released from quarantine, e.g., "sterilized—awaiting test results" or an equivalent designation.

The Contractor agrees to state on the accompanying documents his facility address, signature of the release authority, the device, the supplemental agreement number of sterilization specification number, the number of units, the date and the lot or control numbers.

The Contractor agrees to ship the sterilized devices to the establishment(s) as stated in the supplemental agreement.

Non-Conformance and Corrective Actions

For the pertinent time after shipping the released devices to the Contractor, the Manufacturer agrees to inform the Contractor of any subsequently discovered significant, non-conformance of the device or process related to the ability of the devices to be sterilized without degradation and to specify the disposition of the nonconforming devices. The Manufacturer agrees to take appropriate corrective action before releasing another shipment to the Contractor.

Prior to the release of the sterilized devices, the Contractor agrees to inform the Manufacturer of any significant process or equipment malfunction that may have left or rendered the devices non-sterile or significantly degraded the devices or primary packaging. The Manufacturer will be responsible for the disposition of abnormal findings and will advise the Contractor of the desired resolution within _____ hours.

For the pertinent time after shipping the released devices to the Manufacturer or other designee, the Contractor agrees to inform the Manufacturer of any subsequently discovered non-conformance of the overall sterilization process that may have left or rendered the devices non-sterile or may have significantly degraded the devices or primary packaging. The Contractor agrees to make appropriate corrective action before processing another load for the Manufacturer.

The Manufacturer agrees to inform the Contractor of any significant complaints about distributed devices that are purported to be non-sterile or degraded due to the sterilization process.

Where mutual support is essential, the parties agree to cooperate in executing corrective actions as needed to resolve device or process non-conformance with respect to the agreed upon sterilization specifications.

Outline of Sample for Sterilization with ETO

Specific Device Supplemental Agreement for Contract Sterilization
Supplemental Agreement Number _____

The specific device supplemental agreement is required by the agreement and when all blanks are completed or marked N/A and signed (where indicated) by the Manufacturer and Contractor, it forms a part of the Agreement for Contract Sterilization between the parties.
The specific device and requirements for sterilization are:

Device or Device Family:
Manufacturer's Device Specification Number: Revision:
Validation history record number:

Sterilization Cycle Parameters

Preconditioning cycle: Yes ____ No ____
Humidity: Temperature: Dwell Time:
Chemical Indicator:
Bio-Indicator Type: Population:
Loading and Indicator location pattern number: rev:

1. ___ Preconditioning chamber:
     Humidity: Temperature: Dwell Time:
2. ETO concentration:
3. Diluent Gas:
4. ___ Pressure Cycle:
5. ___ Pre ETO Vac. Cycle:
6. ___ Post ETO Vac. Cycle:
7. ___ Humidity and Dwell:
8. ___ Temp:
9. ___ Exposure Time:
10. ___ Chamber Aeration:

(Note: This educational material is not an official statement binding FDA.)

(Write REC to left of item 1 and items 4 through 10 if the item must be recorded on an instrument chart. (A diagram of the parameter cycle versus time may be used instead of listing the parameters as done in items 1 through 10 above. The diagram must be documented and approved.)

Other Cycle History Records:

Warehouse Aeration Cycle:

BI Disposition:

Device Samples and Disposition:

Device Disposition:

Finished Device History Record & Disposition:

Manufacturer	**Contract Sterilizer**
Address:	Address:
Signature:	Signature:
Date:	Date:

This outline of a sample supplemental agreement for a specific device and process is directed toward sterilization with ETO. It must be rewritten to meet the Manufacturer's and Contract Sterilizer's legal, specific device and specific process requirements (e.g. steam, radiation, dry heat). Complete a separate supplemental agreement each time the device or family of devices requires a different set of sterilization parameters. If only one sterilization process is involved, the supplemental agreement and its attachments such as loading patterns may be a permanent appendix of the main agreement.

Appendix C.4

Application of Medical Device GMPs to Computerized Devices and Manufacturing Processes

November, 1990

Contents

Foreword

In October 1982, the Food and Drug Administration established the Center for Devices and Radiological Health (CDRH) by merging the Bureau of Medical Devices and the Bureau of Radiological Health.

The Center develops and implements national programs to protect the public health in the fields of medical devices and radiological health. These programs are intended to assure the safety, effectiveness, and proper labeling of medical devices, to control unnecessary human exposure to potentially hazardous ionizing and nonionizing radiation, and to ensure the safe, efficacious use of such radiation.

The Center publishes the results of its work in scientific journals and in its own technical reports. These reports provide a mechanism for disseminating results of CDRH and contractor projects. They are sold by the Government Printing Office and/or the National Technical Information Service.

We welcome your comments and requests for further information.

> Walter E. Gundaker
> Acting Director
> Center for Devices and
> Radiological Health

Preface

This document contains general information for applying the Device GMPs to computerized manufacturing processes and to the manufacture of computerized medical devices. It is intended to provide guidance to FDA investigators and supplement document FDA 84-4191, Medical Device GMP Guidance for FDA Investigators.[1]

This document is not intended to suggest that the procedures and practices discussed are the only ones the Food and Drug Administration finds acceptable. Computer technology, as well as the procedures for duplication and evaluation of software, is changing at a fast pace. Therefore, it is the responsibility of the manufacturer to establish procedures and controls adequate to assure compliance with applicable GMP requirements. The adequacy of each manufacturer's practices will be evaluated on a case-by-case basis.

This document is also designed to supplement FDA issued compliance policy statements and reference manuals, such as Compliance Policy Guides,[2] and FDA's Technical Reference on Software Development Activities.[3] These materials should be reviewed in conjunction with this document.

1.0 Purpose

This document outlines GMP requirements as applied to the manufacture of computerized devices and the control of computerized manufacturing and quality assurance systems. It is intended to provide guidance to FDA investigators and to supplement FDA document 84-4191, Medical Device GMP Guidance for FDA Investigators.[1] This document is also designed to supplement FDA issued compliance policy statements and references on Software Development Activities Policy Guides[2] and FDA's Technical Reference on Software Development Activities.[3]

2.0 Scope

This document applies to manufacturers who utilize automated systems for manufacturing, quality assurance, and/or record-keeping. It also applies to manufacturers of medical devices that are driven or controlled by software.

3.0 Introduction

The GMP contains requirements which assure that specifications are established for the device, components, labeling, and packaging and that these specifications are met. The GMP is written in general terms in order that it may apply to a broad diversity of medical devices and manufacturing processes found in the medical device industry. Because of this, FDA investigators sometimes have difficulty in applying the GMP to certain aspects of the industry. Automation is one area where investigators have expressed difficulty in applying the GMP, whether it is automation of individual devices or automation of a manufacturing system.

This document is intended to assist investigators in properly interpreting and applying the GMP to this industry. However, investigators should understand that while the procedures and controls described in this document are acceptable to FDA, they may not be the only procedures and controls acceptable to FDA. Manufacturers are free to use other approaches as long as they can provide assurance that they are adequate in meeting the applicable GMP requirements.

4.0 Application of the GMP

4.1 General

In order to assure that only safe and effective devices are distributed, devices must be designed and manufactured under adequate quality assurance controls. The following is a section-by-section discussion of the GMP as it applies to computers and describes the types of controls that would typically be expected. The actual controls utilized by a manufacturer may differ from those described. When they do, investigators should obtain justification from the manufacturer.

The validity of the manufacturer's approach should be evaluated in terms of the manufacturer's demonstrated degree of success in applying the approach to the manufacture and distribution of only safe and effective devices.

4.2 Organization (820.20)

The GMPs require all manufacturers of medical devices to establish and implement an organizational structure that includes a formal quality assurance program and sufficient personnel to assure that all devices are manufactured in accordance with the GMPs. The program that a manufacturer establishes to implement the GMP requirements effectively becomes the firm's quality assurance program.

In order to comply with the GMP requirements, manufacturers organize themselves in such a way that there is adequate and continuous control over all activities affecting quality. Technical, administrative and human factors affecting quality of the products produced are properly controlled. Such controls are oriented towards the reduction, elimination and prevention of quality deficiencies.

The responsibility, authority and the interrelation of all personnel who manage, perform and verify work affecting quality is defined. The program emphasizes the identification of actual or potential quality problems and the initiation of remedial or preventive measures.

All the elements, requirements and provisions adopted by a company for its quality assurance program are documented in a systematic and orderly manner in the form of written policies and procedures. Such documentation (e.g. quality plans, manuals, records, etc.) ensures a common understanding of quality policies and procedures.

Management assigns an individual the responsibility and authority for ensuring that the requirements of the GMP are implemented and maintained.

Part 820.20(a) contains some specific responsibilities of the QA program.

4.2.1 Quality Assurance Program Requirements (820.20(a))

Part 820.20(a)(1) of the GMP mandates that all production records must be reviewed. This requirement applies equally to manual and computerized records.

Per Part 820.20(a)(2) each manufacturer is responsible for assuring the acceptability of components and labeling, as well as the finished device, regardless of whether they are manufactured in-house or provided under contract by another company (vendor supplied). Therefore, a manufacturer's quality assurance program includes procedures for assuring approval or rejection of contract-supplied software.

To assure that only acceptable software is received, manufacturers who purchase software from vendors establish a program for assuring that the vendor has demonstrated a capability to produce quality software. The program provides assurance that the requirements for the software are clearly defined, communicated and completely understood by the vendor. This may require written procedures for the preparation of requirements and purchase orders, vendor conferences prior to contract release and other appropriate methods. In order to assure understanding, manufacturers establish a close working relationship and feedback system with the vendor. In this way a program of continual quality improvements can be maintained and quality disputes avoided or settled quickly.

Acceptance procedures for contract-supplied software may vary. For example, they may include third-party certification. The finished device manufacturer, however, has the primary responsibility for assuring the software is adequate for its intended use. When third-party certification is used, the certification package includes adequate documented evidence that the software complies with specified requirements. Examples of such evidence include documentation of the review, including procedures used to evaluate the software, the results of the evaluation and evidence of the decision-making process used by the manufacturer to conclude that the software will fulfill its requirements. When the contract-supplied software includes more functions than are utilized, those portions of the program which will be used are evaluated for their application. Also, the software is evaluated to assure the unused portions do no interfere with proper performance. Specific requirements which apply to these activities are covered under 820.80(a), 820.160, and 820.161 and are discussed later in this document.

Part 820.20(a)(3) requires manufacturers to identify quality assurance problems and to verify the implementation of solutions to those problems. Thus, quality data collected by a firm through its various documented process and control systems, such as work operations, processes, quality records, service reports and customer complaints, are evaluated by appropriate methods (e.g., trend analysis) to determine if there are trends or recurring problems which warrant corrective action.

These reviews are an important element of an effective quality assurance program and are important for identifying conditions or situations (e.g., device design problems or problems associated with the manufacturing process) which might not otherwise be apparent or might be dismissed as isolated incidents. The results of investigations and corrective actions are, of course, documented.

Per 820.20(a)(4) all quality assurance checks must be appropriate and adequate for their purpose and must be performed correctly. QA software checks may be *both* quantitative or qualitative; testing is not restricted to quantitative measurements. Testing of software involves evaluation of conformance to specifications and ability to perform as intended. Therefore, test results may vary in expression from a numerical value which is the checksum for the program or the result of a complex mathematical calculation to a qualitative determination, such as the functional adequacy of the illumination of a light or a display.

QA checks of the original program before it is released to manufacturing include review of documentation to assure that the program conforms to its design specifications, which are covered by 820.181(a), as well as an evaluation to assure it performs as intended. It is common for the program to be evaluated as segments or modules first, then as an integrated unit, and finally a system. The documented test results are evidence of the evaluation. When software is involved in manufacturing and quality assurance, evaluation is covered by 820.100(a)(1) and 820.61. This evaluation is performed when software is developed in-house, and, when it has been supplied by a vendor.

After the program has been accepted, and released to production, it is evaluated to assure that it is accurately transferred/copied from storage medium to storage medium (e.g., magnetic disks to integrated electronic circuitry chips). The evaluation also assures that the working master copy remains an exact duplicate of the program that was approved and released to production and

that the software has not undergone unapproved revision or modification.

Section 820.20(b) requires manufacturers to conduct planned
and periodic audits of their quality assurance program. Every quality audit includes a review of procedures and activities to assure
standard operating procedures are adequate and are being followed and that all elements of the quality system are effective in
achieving stated quality objectives. As applied to software, this audit includes evaluation of procedures used to assure that hardware
and software are adequate for their intended use, and that SOPs remain adequate. The audits extend to all phases of software design,
development, testing, design transfer, implementation, and maintenance activities related to computerized processes and devices.

Since in many cases manufacturers rely on suppliers to assure
quality of software, the quality audit includes the supplier. On-site
assessments are made of the supplier's capability to produce quality software and other components.

Audits are conducted by individuals qualified to perform the
task. Evidence is available to show that individuals involved in
software QA review and evaluation have been adequately trained.
As with any other device manufacturing process, these individuals
have a working knowledge of how the device is made, and they
should also have a working knowledge of developing and documenting software.

The results of the audits are documented and brought to the
attention of the personnel responsible for the areas audited and
upper management. Timely corrective action is carried out and
verified as necessary.

4.3 Personnel Training (820.25(a))

All personnel must have adequate training to perform their assigned responsibilities. This means that individuals responsible for
producing and evaluating software have the necessary education,
training, and experience to assure that the software is properly
prepared and maintained. These individuals know how to develop
the software and have an understanding of how to properly document and test the program to minimize, with an adequate degree of
confidence, the effect of latent faults.

Also of concern are the training, experience, and knowledge of
employees responsible for duplicating software and handling magnetic storage media (e.g., floppy disks, tapes, PROM chips, etc.).
Training is conducted to assure these individuals are fully aware of

their responsibilities, particularly of the controls and procedures they must follow to assure that software incorporated into the final medical device is not adversely effected and performs as intended. Appropriate records of training/experience are maintained.

4.4 Environmental Control (820.46)

Where environmental conditions could have an adverse impact on a device's fitness for use, the conditions must be controlled. In general, this applies to the manufacturing environment and areas used for storage of components, and the finished device.

Computers and software storage media may be sensitive to the environment. Mainframe (and some mini-) computers generally call for stringent temperature and humidity controls, and all computers are subject to some degree of environmental limitations.

Overheating, whether from an external source or from the computer's own electronic circuits, can have an adverse effect on a computer's ability to operate properly. Failures caused by system overheating may range from total failure or shutdown of the system to intermittent errors. The maximum temperature at which a microprocessor or central processing unit (CPU) can operate is usually stated in the processor/CPU specifications established by the system's manufacturer.

Humidity may also adversely affect a computer system. Because the computer system is an electronic unit, excessive humidity can have a detrimental effect on electrical contacts and circuitry within the system. Conversely, a dry environment will increase the possibility of static discharges that can damage electrical circuits, software storage components (e.g., chips, and other static sensitive components) and, in turn, have an adverse effect on the software.

The degree of environmental control required is determined by the manufacturer of the finished device. Specifications are developed for the environment and maintained in the device master record. A control system is implemented to assure that the environmental specifications are not exceeded. This environmental control system is periodically inspected for proper functioning and the inspections are documented.

Some electronic hardware components such as computer chips which house the software assembled in the device, are sensitive to electrostatic discharge (ESD). When ESD is a concern, only personnel at properly ESD-controlled work stations handle blank static-sensitive chips, preprogrammed chips, and the circuit boards containing these chips. ESD controls include grounding, humidity control, negative ion generation, etc. The firm's system for controlling ESD is periodically inspected to assure it is exercising adequate control: Are work stations properly grounded? Are employees, working with ESD-sensitive components grounded to work stations? Is humidity monitored? Routine inspections are part of the equipment maintenance procedures.

Other forms of preprogrammed media such as disks (hard and floppy) and magnetic tapes are also handled only in environmentally controlled areas. In areas where these are used, the ability to retrieve data may also be adversely affected by exposure to dust and dirt; therefore, dust and dirt is controlled in addition to ESD.

Components and other media are protected from sources of magnetic interference which can result in the potential accidental erasure of the software by a magnetic field from a permanent magnet or electromagnet. If the product is electromagnetic interference (EMI) sensitive, then efforts to control and/or test for EMI are documented.

4.5 Equipment (820.60)

Section 820.60 of the GMP mandates periodic maintenance of equipment used in the manufacturing process, when applicable. When applied to the software used in production, working master copies of software are periodically challenged and compared against the archived master as a means of assuring that the working copy of the released version is a true copy of the master. Unauthorized changes may compromise the accuracy and reliability of the process.

Comparison of two or more computer programs may be accomplished by a number of different procedures. One common method uses a software utility program which compares two programs and prints differences found between them. A comparison of disk directories between the master and working copies as well as the use of some comparative programs can assist in identifying the differences. The differences may be as simple as one copy containing additional utility programs while the others do not. Another procedure involves comparing the checksums of the preprogrammed chips. The checksum is the value which results from the addition of the values stored in each address on the chip. The values from each chip of the working copy are then compared with the checksums of the archived master. Any difference between the two reflects a discrepancy in the programs and indicates a change in either of the two copies, but it does not identify the location of the difference(s). This is accomplished separately.

Only the current version of software that has been approved and released for use by the device manufacturer is available in the manufacturing/quality control area. When software revisions have been made and released for use, obsolete versions of the program are removed from use. Appropriate corresponding documentation (e.g., written manufacturing procedures and/or design specifications) is also updated and distributed in a timely manner.

A written maintenance procedure is recommended as a dependable means for assuring that all aspects of equipment maintenance are covered.

4.6 Measurement Equipment (820.61)

All computerized production and quality assurance measurement equipment must be suitable for its intended use and capable of producing valid results. To establish confidence in the adequacy of computerized equipment, the hardware (sensors, transmitters, etc.) is calibrated and the software is challenged and validated to assure fitness for its intended use. Calibration is done in accordance with written calibration procedures and schedules. The frequency of calibration may be dependent upon the purpose of the measurement taken, stability, and how often the equipment is used.

Calibration of computer hardware is similar to calibration of any other electromechanical system. The sensor's measurement of temperature, voltage, resistance, etc., is compared against the measurement of a known standard traceable to the National Institute of Standards and Technology (formally the National Bureau of Standards) or other acceptable standard. An important part of the calibration activity is to assure that measurements are properly transmitted across computer communication lines and properly interpreted by the computer system.

Verification of properly transmitted measurements is accomplished by comparing the measured value that has been input into the computer system with the value of the traceable standard.

The PROM programmer, a piece of manufacturing equipment, is used for programming integrated circuits (ICs). To assure that integrated circuits are adequately programmed, equipment maintenance and calibration need for programmers should be considered, including proper voltage, current, and pulse shape.

Modification of the hardware and/or configuration of the system may require system recalibration. Procedures for handling modifications are addressed in standard operating procedures.

When automated production or QA systems are used, the software programs are validated. Validation of system software is a complex activity which must be carefully planned and performed, before use of the software package, and after significant revision of the system occurs. Validation may also be required after any revision of the operating system software. Software verification and validation activities are discussed in greater detail in FDA's reference manual, *Software Development Activities.*[3]

4.7 Components (820.80)

The GMP regulation requires that manufacturers establish adequate procedures for acceptance and storage of components to assure that only those components that are acceptable for use are released to manufacturing.

4.7.1 Acceptance of Components (820.80(a))

The components of a software driven device typically consist of circuit boards, resistors, transistors, and other discrete items commonly found in electrical devices. However, there are two additional components of special concern in a software driven device: the actual software that controls functions of the device and the hardware on which the software is stored or mounted.

Software inspection and testing are normally accomplished in a manner different from that performed on the discrete components of the device. The component specifications for software are usually referred to as the software requirements. These include user or device requirements (e.g., the device will respond in a specific manner to a specific input), and they also cover system requirements which are functions associated with the internal workings of, or handling of, data by the software. System requirements may include functions such as error checking, polling, fault tolerance, etc. Ability of the software to meet both user and system requirements is crucial to proper operation of the device.

Preparation and use of an adequate test plan, based on knowledge of software logic and the hardware environment in which the software will run, will assure that software is adequately tested or evaluated, and thereby establish confidence that it does meet specifications. In most cases, evaluation of the software requires not only testing separately from the device by simulation testing (which may use a database with known inputs) but also by testing it in the environment in which it will be used (i.e., the finished device). For example, a database which includes signals of ventricular fibrillation may be used to evaluate one function of a cardiac monitor. Because of the complexity of both software and hardware, this testing may be performed as part of the manufacturer's software development and software quality assurance activities. these tests are routinely referenced as software verification and validation. Final versions of approved test procedures for the software and results of the final tests document that acceptance criteria have been met.

After it is determined that the software is acceptable for use, consideration is given to the need for periodic retests. Retests are usually necessary when the software (operating system or application program) is revised or a software failure is encountered.

When preprogrammed storage media such as chips, disks, etc., are received as components, acceptance procedures assure that software contained in these components is the current version and that it has been adequately duplicated. Acceptance evaluation can be accomplished in a number of ways. One method is a bit-by-bit comparison of the software program in the incoming component against a known correct master copy of the program. Another method consists of determining the checksum of the software in the incoming component and comparing it against the known checksum for the current version of the program. (This test method has been previously discussed in the "Equipment" section of this document; however, the method is also applicable to acceptance of components.) These tests only assure accuracy of the reproduction efforts; they do not reflect the quality of the software program, which can only be determined through the verification and validation test efforts previously discussed.

Incoming acceptance procedures for unprogrammed (blank) ICs vary. They may consist of electrical tests or only a visual examination, depending upon whether history has demonstrated that the supplier can consistently provide a quality product.

Some medical device manufacturers may purchase OEM (Original Equipment Manufacture) products such as CRTs, computers, etc., and combine these products into a medical device system. These may be considered components rather than finished devices. In such cases, it is the medical device manufacturer's responsibility to assure the OEM products are acceptable for use. This may include testing the products individually and as part of the finished system to assure they conform to specifications.

4.7.2   Storage and Handling of Components (820.80(b))

As with all finished device components, software must be adequately identified to prevent mix-up and adequately stored to prevent damage.

Software contained on media such as disks, etc., is identified by providing name or title and version or revision level of the software. This serves to prevent use of obsolete versions of the program.

Programmed media can be damaged by the environment. For example, it is possible that software may be accidentally altered if the hardware which contains the software program is exposed to electrostatic discharge (ESD), or to ultraviolet radiation. Therefore, manufacturers exercise care in the handling and storage of magnetic media and programmed chips. (ESD control has already been covered in this document under 4.4 *Environmental Control* (820.46)).

Employees engaged in handling ESD sensitive components are properly trained and made aware of the results of improper performance or poor ESD control practices.

Electrostatic sensitive chips are stored in ESD protective carriers before they are assembled into circuit boards. Under some conditions, materials promoted for ESD control can actually contribute to ESD. Therefore, materials used are qualified for their use to assure adequacy. Circuit boards containing these components are also protected against ESD damage. It is also important that preprogrammed chips and circuit boards that contain preprogrammed chips be handled only by properly trained personnel at properly ESD controlled work stations.

Some hardware components, whose software can be erased by ultraviolet light, require a protective covering over the erasing "window" of the component. If the window is left uncovered, the program contained on the component may possibly "fade" in time through exposure to fluorescent light, sunlight, or other sources of UV radiation. Protective covers may include a special plastic cap or a piece of light resistant tape placed over the window.

As previously described under 4.4 *Environmental Control* (820.46), exposure to dust or dirt may affect the ability of preprogrammed magnetic media, such as disks or tape, to record and read data. Contents of the disk or tape may also be altered if stored in the vicinity of a strong magnetic field. Therefore, these media are protected from rough handling and temperature extremes, as well as magnetic fields and electromagnetic radiation.

4.8 Critical Devices, Components (820.81)

In addition to the requirements of 820.80 as described above, additional controls are established and implemented for handling critical components of a critical device. Section 820.81(a) requires that specific controls be in place for the acceptance of critical components. Computer components such as integrated circuits (ICs) may be identified as critical components when they are used in a critical device. The complexity of these components can make it difficult for the device manufacturer to adequately test these components for acceptance. In this situation, the device manufacturer may have to rely on the component manufacturer to certify in writing that the required specifications have been met, and require the component manufacturer to provide actual test data. A vendor QA program (as discussed on page 206) is also established to assure confidence in the data.

GMP section 820.81(b) requires that, where possible, the finished device manufacturer must obtain a written agreement from the supplier of critical components which states that the device manufacturer will be notified of any proposed change in a critical component. In relation to computerized devices, this section applies to both hardware and software components that are critical. Hardware may include custom designed components such as gate arrays, programmable logic arrays, ROMs, and analog arrays which may have been made specifically to the finished device manufacturer's specifications. Critical component software may include programs which perform and control critical functions of a device. Whether the components are customized hardware or are a software program, it is important that the finished device manufacturer know when the component supplier makes any changes because a change to a component may adversely impact the finished device.

4.9 Manufacturing Specifications and Processes (820.100)

Specifications and procedures for manufacturing a device must be established, implemented and controlled to assure that the device conforms to its original design or to any approved changes in that design (820.100).

Section 820.100(a)(1) requires all manufacturers to assure that design requirements are properly translated into device and component specifications which are used in production. When applied to computerized operations, this means that manufacturers are prepared to provide evidence that the software used for duplicating the device software and the software used in automated manufacturing or quality assurance meets the software design specifications.

This section is interpreted by FDA to include process validation. When a manufacturing process is automated, the computerized system is validated to assure it performs as intended. In validating computerized equipment, parameters that the system is designed to measure, record, and/or control are evaluated by an independent method until it is demonstrated that the computer system will function properly in its intended environment.

When a manufacturing process is controlled by computer, functional evaluation of the control system may include, but is not limited to, the following activities:

- equipment (peripherals, etc.) and sensor checks using known inputs, which may consist of processing test or simulated data;

- alarm checks at, within, and beyond their operational limits; and,

- evaluation of operator override mechanisms for how they are used by operators and how they are documented.

In case of system failure, evaluations would include:

- how data is updated when in manual operation;

- what happens to data "in process" when the system shuts down;

- what procedures are in place to handle system shutdown; and,

- how product or information handled by the computerized process is affected.

Process validation is conducted to evaluate the effectiveness and repeatability of the process and its impact on the device during both expected operation and worst case situations. When software is involved, this activity may in many cases have to be accomplished in two steps: first, the software is integrated into the system and the system is evaluated independently of the system it is to control; second, the software is integrated into the system and the system is evaluated.

Section 820.100(a)(2) requires that changes to specifications of a device, which includes software specifications, must be subject to controls as stringent as those applied to the original software program. Usually, this means validation that includes an evaluation of how the change impacts on the rest of the software. For example, if the addition of a subroutine or function is determined to have little effect on the device or process, only a limited number of modules may require retesting and revalidation. On the other hand, changes such as updating the operating system software could have an impact on the entire application software, thereby requiring more intensive evaluation. In any event, all changes are evaluated to assure that they are appropriate (that they achieve their intended purpose) and that they do not adversely affect the unchanged software.

Revisions to software follow established change control procedures to assure that the history of the changes are maintained and that each change is properly reviewed, approved and dated before implementation.

In order to control and maintain the software and to know its configuration at any time, documented evidence is needed to demonstrate why each change was made, that each change is adequate, and that it has been approved for use. As with any device, this information is essential for investigating device defects.

Also, if the change significantly extends the indication for use, or affects the safety or effectiveness of the device, a new 510(k) or PMA supplement may need to be submitted to FDA. If the change is made to correct a problem with respect to safety, effectiveness or performance, a recall may be needed.

4.9.1 Processing Controls (820.100(b))

When the possibility exists for the device to deviate from its design specifications as a result of an inadequately controlled manufacturing process, written manufacturing procedures must be established. As applied to software, this GMP provision includes the process of duplicating the currently released, approved "master" software program onto other storage media, generally for assembly into the device. To assure that this process is adequate and produces consistent results, manufacturers have established written procedures.

Standard operating procedures (SOPs) for software handling and duplication are controlled documents. Any changes or revisions made in these documents are subjected to formal review and approval by designated individual(s) before implementation. Once approved, the revised procedures are conveyed to appropriate personnel in a timely manner.

Process controls also include computer security and may involve limiting physical access to the computer on which the software is written and/or tested and also may include limiting access to the software itself to prevent unauthorized changes. Software security may include the use of passwords, passkeys, etc. Assignment and use of these security measures should also be controlled.

4.10   Finished Device Inspection (820.160)

Adequate procedures must be in place and implemented to assure that the finished device meets its design specifications. Testing should verify that the software functions utilized perform as intended and that unused functions do not adversely affect performance. For software driven devices, it is sometimes impossible to fully qualify the computer program through performance of function tests. Because of the computer program's logic and branching capabilities, a specific task performed by the device may be accomplished in one manner, one time, and depending on the logic of the program and the data entered, in a totally different manner another time. Therefore, independent testing of the software itself is conducted if the true capabilities and limitations of the device and software are to be known. This was discussed earlier in the "Components" section of this document. Rarely can the full functional capabilities of the software be demonstrated by testing only the finished device.

Therefore, once the software has been accepted as a component for use, the adequate control of the duplication process during manufacturing has been established through validation and process control, it is usually not necessary to re-verify performance of software in each unit, batch, or lot of devices manufactured. Instead, assurance is established that the correct version of the software program is included with the device. One way to do this is to access the program and call up its current revision or version identification either on a visual display or a printout. This method, however, is not always possible. A second method consists of verifying that the labels on the program chips or magnetic media reflect the proper software revision level identified in the device master record (DMR).

Finished product inspection of a software driven medical device also includes tests normally associated with an electromechanical device. Although these tests may not fully challenge the software, they help to assure that the device has been properly assembled.

4.11 Failure Investigation (820.162)

When failure occurs in a distributed software driven device or in a distributed device which consists solely of software, an adequate investigation must be conducted to identify the cause. For example, in a software driven device, the failure may be related to the device design, the manufacturing process, or the quality assurance equipment used in the evaluation of the device. In a device that consists only of software, the cause of the failure may be related to the software design or the process used for duplicating the software. When the failure of a finished device is attributable to the software used in manufacturing or quality assurance, identification of the cause of a failure may require review of the software program's logic and of the test procedures and results, as well as a retesting of the program. Further reviews may be required of the duplication process and of environmental control records for those areas where ESD sensitive components were handled and assembled.

If the software error is in the device, similar investigative activities are conducted. In either situation, the investigation extends to determining effects on other products, and results in a written record of the investigation and any follow-up action and corrective action taken.

4.12 Records, General Requirements (820.180)

Recordkeeping requirements that apply to nonautomated devices also apply to software controlled devices. Records must be available for review and copying by FDA employees, including those records which have been computerized and placed on computer storage media such a magnetic tape, disks, etc.

All records maintained in accordance with 21 CFR 820 are required to be retained for a period of time equivalent to the design and expected life of the device, but in no case less than two years from the date of release of the device for commercial distribution.

4.13 Device Master Record (820.181)

The device master record (DMR) consists of diagrams, descriptions, schematics, etc., that constitute the specifications for the medical device product, the manufacturing process, and QA program. In addition to items detailing specifications for the device hardware, the device master record for a software driven product also includes detailed specifications for the device software. Detailed specifications are also required when the device consists of only software.

All records and documents contained in the device master record are controlled documents, including documentation related to software. Any revision or change of the software program or its supporting documentation are made in accordance with formal change control procedures and authorized by signature of the designated individual(s). Magnetically coded badges and other electronic identifiers may be used in lieu of signatures if adequate controls are in place to prevent their misuse.

4.13.1   Specifications (820.181(a))

The device master record must include specifications for the device. When software is part of the device, specifications include or refer to:

- the final, complete, approved software design requirements, which describe in narrative and/or pictorial form, such as a flow chart, what the software is intended to do (e.g., to control or monitor something) and how it will accomplish these tasks. Also included is a description of how the software will interact with the hardware to accomplish various functions of the device's design. The specifications may also include a checksum for the program. The description is in a form that can be understood by all individuals who work on and/or will maintain the program during its life. Note that the description does not include documentation of the working drafts (or in-process steps) of the software design; it only includes the final approved specifications. The procedures for evaluation of the software to assure specifications are met are covered by 820.181(c).

- a description of the device's computer hardware system specifications, such as interfaces, connections, and media for storage of the program in the device.

- the computer source code as either hard copy or on magnetic medium. It usually is necessary for the finished device manufacturer to have the source code. This documentation is indispensable for adequately maintaining the program and evaluating the impact of any change on the rest of the program.

  It is important that the device manufacturer collaborate with the software vendor in the initial stages when software specifications are being developed and when any changes are introduced in order to assure that the intent of the design is adequately translated into software code. In these situations, the device manufacturer and software vendor establishes a contract that delineates responsibilities relating to the development and maintenance of the software.

The program source code typically includes or refers to adequate documentation which describes the subroutines or modules for the language used. Additional documentation that describes the design of the program is maintained. The intent is to assure that individuals maintaining the program have sufficient documentation to fully understand the purpose of the software design. Depth and detail of the documentation are proportionate to the complexity of the systems involved.

4.13.2 Production Process Procedures (820.181(b))

The DMR must contain production process specifications. When applied to software controlled processes the DMR includes procedures for environmental control and specifications where applicable; procedures for duplication of software for assembly into the finished device; specifications for use of any automated or computerized manufacturing equipment or processes; and specifications for any computerized packaging and labeling operations. The DMR also includes procedures for computer/software security, if implemented.

To assure consistency of results, the DMR includes written change control procedures and any change in software that is part of the device or that is used in manufacturing or in quality assurance.

4.13.3   Quality Assurance Procedures and Specifications (820.181(c))

The DMR must also include all documentation used to determine quality of conformance to established specifications for the components, device, packaging, labeling and manufacturing processes. For software, this includes, but is not limited to, identification of any automated test equipment, as well as test procedures and criteria used to evaluate the current device software program for acceptance for use in manufacturing (820.80(a)) and for acceptance of hardware components used to store the software in the device (also 820.80(a)). For computerized manufacturing processes, this also includes any tests which are performed to evaluate the adequacy of the process, such as evaluating the integrity of package seals and verifying that the correct label was applied.

4.13.4   Labeling (820.181(d))

The final element required by the device master record concerns labeling for the finished medical device. Because of the possible complexity of a software driven device, extensive labeling may be required for adequate user instructions. This labeling may take the form of user manuals or it may be embedded directly into the software for the device, appearing on screen as instructions and menus.

User manuals or directions are written in clearly understood terminology and consist of operating instructions that explain how the system works and the procedures to be followed. Manuals include an explanation of all advisories, alarm and error messages, as well as corrective actions to be taken when these situations occur.

4.14   Device History Record (820.184)

The device history record (DHR) demonstrates that the device is manufactured in accordance with the specifications in the device master record. This agreement is shown by documented evidence that manufacturing and test procedures have been followed and that the results meet acceptance criteria. When software is part of the device, this documentation includes a record of the version of the software which was assembled into the device, results from evaluating the device software (e.g., performance), in addition to all documentation needed to show that the software was adequately reproduced during manufacturing.

Adequate production records are in place to properly document all significant activities. For example, software that is part of a device may be copied into components, such as PROMs (Programmable Read Only Memory Chips), which are then assembled into the device. Production records for this activity document the results of the duplication process. For example, when checksums are used to identify the revision of the software which is duplicated into components, the production record documents the checksum and the number of components which were copied as well as the date the activity was performed. All production records are included in, or referred to in, the device history record.

4.15   Critical Devices, Automated Data Processing (820.195)

Section 820.195 applies only to manufacturing or quality assurance activities associated with critical devices. Automated data processing is the means used to gather and analyze information on some characteristic of the device manufacturing process or QA program without direct use of an operator to control the activity or verify the results. Automated data processing systems provide an effective method for performing routine, repetitive tasks. Although generally more reliable than manual equivalents, such systems demand adequate controls for equipment setup and programming. The GMP regulation requires a manufacturer to implement controls that will assure the correctness and appropriateness of these programs, program changes, equipment and data input and output.

4.16   Complaint Files (820.198)

Firms must prepare and implement adequate complaint handling systems including the review, investigation, and evaluation of both hardware and software failures of distributed devices. A notation in the complaint file that a system has failed as a result of a software error is supported with data or evidence to justify that conclusion. When a software failure is encountered, an investigation is conducted to determine the cause of the error and its impact on the capabilities of the device and similar devices.

Many manufacturers use computers for recording and tracking complaint information contained in paper documents, such as letters from complainants or laboratory reports. The complete information may be copied into the computer system in lieu of maintaining the original documents. If the documents are retained, however, the computerized complaint record makes reference to corresponding paperwork.

Complaints are an excellent source of information about device design and the manufacturing process by which the device was produced. When complaint files are computerized, a software program that provides a means of determining the existence of any similar recurring problems with the device, similar devices, or with the manufacturing process, which might indicate a need for possible corrective action, is invaluable.

—END—

Appendix A: Definitions

Archived Master (copy of software)	A software library which contains formally approved and released versions of software and documentation from which copies are made.
Checksum	The value from adding the individual values at each address of the hardware component which contains the software program. This value may also be used to indicate software versions.
Chips	An electronic hardware component consisting of integrated microcircuits which perform a significant number of functions.
Disk Directories	Index of the file names on the disk. It may also include file size, date of creation, and date last altered.
Electrostatic Discharge (ESD)	A discharge of the potential energy that electric charges possess by virtue of their positions relative to each other. This discharge may adversely affect hardware sensitive to potential differences.

Error Checking	A means of determining if recording of data, its input into a computer system, and its transfer within the system, including transmission, is correct.
Fault Tolerance	Systems that continue to operate satisfactorily in the presence of faults (i.e., hardware failures).
Integrated Circuits (IC)	Complex electronic circuits etched on small semiconductor chips.
Master Copies of Software	The approved versions of the software from which copies are made for use and reproduction in the manufacturing environment.
Polling	In a data communications system, a line control method in which the computer asks each terminal on the system, in turn, if it has a message to send.
Programmable Read Only Memory Chips (PROMS)	Memory chips of which the contents can be read but not altered during program execution. However, the contents of the memory can be altered before it is assembled in the computer system.
PROM Programmer	Electronic equipment which is used to transfer a software program into a PROM.
Third-Party Certification	The procedure and action, by a duly authorized independent body, of confirming that a system, software subsystem, or computer program is capable of satisfying its specified requirements in an operational environment. Certification usually takes place in the field under actual or simulated operational conditions, and is used to evaluate the software itself and the specifications to which the software was designed. Certification activities take place under a written, approved (by the manufacturer) protocol.
Validation	Establishing documented evidence which provides a high degree of assurance that a specific process will consistently produce a product meeting its predetermined specifications and quality attributes.

Validation Testing	Testing that commences after the completion of the development testing and includes module and subsystem level testing. These tests can be considered to be "rehearsals;" they are basically gross tests of the coding against specifications.
Verification	The process of reviewing, inspecting, testing, checking, auditing, or otherwise establishing and documenting whether or not items, processes, services, or documents conform to specified requirements.
Verification Testing	An acceptance test of software. These tests are rigorous and detailed and will result in the software quality certification that the coding is in complete agreement with the specifications, design, and test documentation.
Worst Case	A set of conditions encompassing upper and lower processing limits and circumstances, including those within standard operating procedures, which pose the greatest chance of process or product failure when compared to ideal conditions. Such conditions do not necessarily induce product or process failure.

Appendix B: References

1. FDA 84-4191: Medical Device GMP Guidance for FDA Investigators (April 1984).

2. FDA Compliance Policy Guides

   Office of Enforcement, Compliance Policy Guide 7132A.07: Computerized Drug Processing: Input/Output Checking (October 1, 1982).

   Office of Enforcement, Compliance Policy Guide 7132A.08: Computerized Drug Processing; Identification of "Persons" on Batch Production and Control Records, (December 1, 1982).

Office of Enforcement, Compliance Policy Guide 7132A.11: Computerized Drug Processing; CGMP Applicability to Hardware and Software, (December 1, 1984).

Office of Enforcement, Compliance Policy Guide 7132A.12: Computerized Drug Processing; Vendor Responsibility, (January 18, 1985).

Office of Enforcement, Compliance Policy Guide 7132A.15: Computerized Drug Processing; Source Code for Process Control Application Programs, (April 16, 1987).

3. FDA 84-4191: Software Development Activities, Reference Materials and Training Aids for Investigators (July 1987).

4. FDA Field Computer Specialists and their location: Martin Browning, DFI/ORA, Rockville, MD; John Kunkel, Minneapolis District; Philip Piasecki, Boston District; Sam Clark, Atlanta District; Paul Figarole, Baltimore District; Dwight Herd, San Juan District.

5. References for Definitions:

    Capron, H.L. and Williams, Brian K., *Computers and Data Processing,* 1982, The Benjamin/Cummings Publishing Company, Inc.

    Parker, Sybil P., Editor-in-Chief, *McGraw-Hill Dictionary of Scientific and Technical Terms,* 1984, McGraw-Hill Book Company.

    Ralston, Anthony, Editor, *Encyclopedia of Computer Science and Engineering,* 1983, Van Nostrand Reinhold Company.

    Foster, Richard A., *Introduction to Software Quality Assurance,* 1975, R. A. Foster.

    Dersey, Roger M., *Digital Circuits and Devices,* 1985, John Wiley and Sons, Inc.

    Fraf, Rudolf F., *Modern Dictionary of Electronics,* 1977, Howard W. Sams and Company, Inc.

    Jay, Frank, Editor-in-Chief, *IEEE Standard Dictionary of Electrical and Electronics Terms,* 1984, The Institute of Electrical and Electronics Engineers, Inc.

6. Recommended References:

FDA 87-4179: CDRH, Device Good Manufacturing Practices Manual, 4th Edition, Division of Small Manufacturers Assistance, OTA (November 1987).

FDA Compliance Program Guidance Manual, Compliance Program 7382.830, Inspection of Medical Device Manufacturers (October 1985).

Center for Drugs and Biologics and Center for Devices and Radiological Health, Guideline on General Principles of Process Validation (May 1987).

FDA 90-4236: CDRH, Preproduction Quality Assurance Planning; Recommendations for Medical Device Manufacturers, Office of Compliance and Surveillance, Division of Compliance Programs (September 1989).

Appendix C.5

Guideline for the Manufacture of In Vitro Diagnostic Products

Food and Drug Administration
Center for Devices and Radiological Health
Office of Compliance

January 10, 1994

Preface

The Food and Drug Administration (FDA) often formulates and disseminates guidelines about matters which are authorized by the laws enforced by the Agency. Accordingly, FDA is making available this guideline. This guideline is intended to be used in conjunction with the current Good Manufacturing Practice (CGMP) regulation (§21 CFR 820); the Labeling for In Vitro Diagnostic Products regulation (§21 CFR 809.10), and the "Guideline on General Principles of

Process Validation." It is also intended to be used in conjunction with the interpretations published in the "Device Good Manufacturing Practices Manual," "Medical Device GMP Guidance for FDA Investigators Manual," and the "GMP Workshop Manual for Sterile Medical Devices."

The notice of availability of the draft guideline stated that it would be issued under §21 CFR 10.90(b), which provides for the use of guidelines to establish procedures or standards of general applicability that are not legal requirements but that are acceptable to the Agency. The Agency is now in the process of considering whether to revise §21 CFR 10.90(b). Although that decision making process is not yet complete, the Agency has decided to publish this guideline. However, this notice and the final guideline are not being issued under the authority of §21 CFR 10.90(b), and the final guideline, although called a guideline, does not operate to bind FDA or any other person in any way.

The Agency advises that this final guideline represents its current position on the requirements of the CGMP regulations for in vitro diagnostic products. The guideline may be useful to manufacturers of in vitro diagnostic products. A person may also choose to use alternate procedures even though they are not provided for in the guideline. If a person chooses to depart from the practices and procedures set forth in the final guideline, that person may wish to discuss the matter further with the Agency to prevent an expenditure of money and effort on activities that may later be determined to be unacceptable by FDA. This guideline does not bind the Agency, and it does not create or confer any rights, privileges, or benefits for or on any person.

Contents

1.0   Scope

In vitro diagnostic products (IVDs), as defined in §21 CFR 809.3(a), are those reagents, instruments, and systems intended for use in the diagnosis of disease or other conditions including a determination of the state of health, in order to cure, mitigate, treat, or prevent disease or its sequelae. Such products are intended for use in the collection, preparation, and examination of specimens taken from the human body. These products are devices as defined in Section 201(h) of the Federal Food, Drug, and Cosmetic Act (the Act), and may also be biological products subject to Section 351 of the Public Health Service Act.

This guideline is applicable to manufacturers of all in vitro diagnostic reagents and systems, but is not intended to apply to manufacturers of IVD instrumentation. As such, this guideline applies to clinical chemistry and clinical toxicology devices, hematology and pathology devices, and immunology and microbiology devices.

This guideline provides general guidance on the application of the medical device good manufacturing practice (GMP) regulation, §21 CFR Part 820, to processes commonly used in the manufacture of IVDs. It includes methods and procedures for meeting requirements of the medical device GMP regulation. It also provides general guidance on the application of the labeling regulation, §21 CFR 809.10, for these devices. This guideline will be used as a reference by FDA investigators during GMP inspections of manufacturer's facilities. When manufacturers elect not to rely upon this guideline, FDA expects that their choice of procedures and processes will be equivalent to ensure the safety and effectiveness of their IVDs.

This guideline has been issued to address several areas concerning the application of the GMP regulation to IVDs. Foremost, the guideline will assist IVD manufacturers in complying with the GMP regulation and also help ensure uniform application of the GMP regulation by FDA. It is understood that this guideline is an attempt to reduce instances of failure to comply with the GMP regulation as reflected in FDA's experience with legal actions, recalls, results of GMP inspections, and data from the Center for Devices and Radiological Health (CDRH) Device Experience Network (DEN). The importance of GMP compliance for IVDs was expressed by the Microbiology Device Classification Panel which agreed to down classify microbiological culture media from Class II (performance standards) to Class I (general controls) dependent on vigorous implementation of the GMP regulation.

2.0   Introduction

The reliability of IVDs is important for accurate diagnosis of a disease or condition and for patient management. Some uses of these products include: diagnosis, screening, therapeutic drug monitoring, collecting epidemiological information, monitoring a course of disease, and antimicrobial susceptibility testing. The failure of an IVD to function as intended, or as stated in the labeling, may result in misdiagnosis and subsequent incorrect, insufficient, unnecessary, or delayed treatment. Consequences to the patient may vary from minimal or nonexistent to serious or life threatening, depending on various factors including the patient's condition and the clinical significance of the diagnostic test. One aspect of the significance or "clinical value" of a specific diagnostic test is whether it is the major means of diagnosis, or whether it is used in conjunction with, or confirmed by, other diagnostic tests along with a physician's evaluation of patient symptoms. A diagnostic test is typically the sole method of diagnosis only when there are no other symptoms or conditions to assist in diagnosis.

IVD reagents and systems include those used in hospitals, clinical laboratories, satellite medical facilities, physician's offices, and in the home by consumers. Depending on the type of facility where a test is performed, the user may or may not have training in laboratory methods and techniques.

3.0　Application of the Regulations to IVDs

The requirements for manufacturers of IVDs are described in §21 CFR 809. The special labeling requirements for these products are identified in Subpart B—Labeling, §21 CFR 809.10. These labeling regulations also specify the stability study and expiration dating requirements for IVDs. Manufacturers must also comply with Subpart C—Requirements for Manufacturers and Producers, §21 CFR 809.20. This subpart requires compliance with the GMP regulation found in Part 820. IVDs are required to be manufactured in accordance with all applicable GMP requirements.

The medical device GMP regulation is an umbrella regulation covering all devices, unless exempted. The GMP regulation specifies quality assurance objectives and principles rather than exact methods, because not all methods are applicable to all processes. It is left to the judgment of each manufacturer to develop methods appropriate to their specific devices and manufacturing processes. To assist manufacturers in developing appropriate methods, this guideline will identify some of the controls implemented for IVDs to ensure the suitability of the product for its labeled and/or intended uses. These are by no means the only controls that may be used to comply with the GMP regulation. IVD manufacturers may use any appropriate method of manufacturing to ensure the quality of IVDs, as long as they have demonstrated by validation that the methods are suitable for their products.

3.1 Product and Process Specifications

There are a number of sections of the GMP that require manufacturers to establish product and process specifications. Section 820.100 requires that written manufacturing specifications and processing procedures be established, implemented, and controlled to assure that the IVD conforms to its original design or any approved changes in that design. Section 820.100(a)(1) of the GMP regulation requires that manufacturers of medical devices establish specifications for all devices, including the components, packaging, and labeling. Section 820.100(b) requires that where deviations from device specifications could occur as a result of the manufacturing process itself, there are written procedures describing any processing controls necessary to assure conformance to specifications. Section 820.181(a) requires that the device master record contain device specifications including appropriate drawings, composition, formulation, and component specifications. Section 820.181(b) requires production process specifications including the appropriate equipment specifications, production methods, production procedures, and production environment specifications. Section 820.181(c) requires quality assurance procedures and specifications including the quality assurance checks used and the quality assurance apparatus used. Section 820.181(d) requires packaging and labeling specifications including the methods and processes used. The following is a means of complying with these GMP sections for establishing product and process specifications for IVDs.

An IVD is typically defined during the preproduction process. Some parameters considered are physical, chemical composition, and microbiological characteristics. Performance characteristics such as accuracy, precision, specificity, and sensitivity are also considered. Once the IVD is properly defined, the parameters and characteristics are translated into written specifications.

These established specifications will determine the appropriate production and process controls such as mixing and filling processes, sterilization, or lyophilization needed to manufacture the IVD. The specifications established for the IVD will also determine the appropriate environmental controls needed, in conjunction with the manufacturing process, to ensure that product specifications are consistently met.

The specifications for the product, the manufacturing process, and the environment are maintained as part of the device master record (DMR), as required by § 820.181.

3.1.1 Product Specifications

Parameters typically considered for IVDs are the product's physical characteristics, chemical composition, microbiological quality, and performance characteristics. This section focuses on two of these, performance characteristics and microbiological characteristics, and provides a means of defining these product specifications.

Performance characteristics define analytical performance, and include characteristics such as accuracy, precision, sensitivity, specificity, purity, and identity. The consistency of these product attributes is not "tested into" the finished product, but is achieved through the establishment of adequate product specifications; and by ensuring that these specifications are met through product and process design, process validation, process water controls, manufacturing controls, and finished product testing.

Microbiological quality for IVDs can be classified into three major categories: *IVDs which are sterile; IVDs which are microbiologically controlled;* and, *IVDs which are microbiologically uncontrolled.*

IVDs are labeled as sterile if sterility of the product is needed for performance, effectiveness, and/or reliability. The product specifications for sterile IVDs include the sterility assurance level (SAL) necessary for the product.

At the other end of the spectrum are IVDs which are microbiologically uncontrolled. These are IVDs which contain components that are either toxic to microorganisms or do not support the growth of microorganisms. Even though microorganisms do not live or multiply in the IVD, the remains or byproducts of any microorganisms are shown not to adversely affect product performance.

Between the two extremes are IVDs that support microorganism life and growth, and the IVD may contain levels of microorganisms. During the preproduction process, a determination is made as to whether these levels could adversely affect product performance. A determination is also made as to whether a certain type (genus, species) of microorganism can adversely affect product performance. Whether the remains (cell walls) or byproducts (biochemicals) of these microorganisms can adversely affect product performance is also determined. When the IVD is stored and used, according to its labeling, and product performance is found to be adversely affected by certain levels, certain types, remains, or byproducts of microorganisms; then, specifications are established to limit the microorganisms to a level that will not have an adverse impact on product performance. In cases where adequate preproduction design has not been performed for this category of IVDs, a retrospective study using adequate information such as product test data, complaint file analysis, trend analysis, bioburden studies, and process control data, along with an examination of the buildings, equipment, employee technique, and clothing requirements, may be capable of showing whether the presence of microorganisms in the IVD can or cannot adversely affect product performance.

The July 1988 document titled "Microbial Load Considerations for Prepared Culture Media Products" prepared jointly by the Health Industry Manufacturers Association (HIMA) and the Association of Microbiological Diagnostics Manufacturers (AMDM) contains applicable supplemental information*(1)*. This document focuses primarily on tissue culture and microbiological media.

3.1.2   Process Specifications

As stated previously, the important characteristics for IVDs are the product's chemical composition, microbiological quality, and its physical and performance characteristics. This section focuses on microbiological characteristics for IVDs and provides a means of defining process specifications.

Appropriate process specifications are established to ensure that IVDs which are labeled sterile are indeed manufactured under appropriate conditions and controls which will result in a sterile product. Sterile IVDs may be produced by either terminal sterilization or by aseptic processing which may include filtration and/or the use of microbiological inhibitory systems. A sterility assurance level (SAL) commensurate with the need for safe and effective performance of the IVD is established as part of the process specifications. A well designed and established manufacturing process is capable of achieving a SAL of at least 10^{-3} for aseptically filled products and at least 10^{-6} for terminally sterilized products. However, a SAL of 10^{-6} may not be appropriate for some terminally sterilized products which are heat labile and where product performance would be adversely affected.

Appropriate process specifications are established to ensure that microbiologically uncontrolled IVDs are manufactured under appropriate conditions and controls which will result in a product which consistently meets all of its specifications. Normally, the process conditions and controls for this category of IVDs are less stringent than those for IVDs which are labeled as sterile and for microbiologically controlled IVDs. These IVDs require minimal or no specific microbiological controls during processing. Filtration or other processes may be employed to ensure an aesthetically acceptable product. Nevertheless, process conditions and controls, along with adequate specifications, are established.

Appropriate process specifications are established to ensure that microbiologically controlled IVDs are manufactured under appropriate conditions and controls which will result in a product which consistently meets all its specifications. A microbiological assurance level (MAL) commensurate with the need for safe and effective performance of the IVD is established as part of the specifications. A well designed and established manufacturing process is capable of achieving a specified MAL. A MAL is specified for each product which, if exceeded, would adversely affect product performance.

Microbiological control is accomplished by filtration, by using preservatives, and/or by implementing appropriate process controls:

A) Some IVDs are filtered to remove certain, but not necessarily all, microorganisms, and testing assures that these specified microorganisms have been removed from the final product. Finished product testing provides reasonable assurance that the presence of other microorganisms will not adversely affect patient sample test results, and that the IVD will perform in a safe (from the user's perspective) and effective (from the patient's perspective) manner. These IVDs may be labeled as "filtered," "sterile filtered," and "sterilized by filtration." (Refer to Appendix II, Definitions).

B) Some IVDs contain low levels of microorganisms which are controlled through the use of microbiological inhibitory systems such as antibiotics, preservatives, pH control, or antisera. When preservatives or antibiotics are used, known amounts are added which effectively inhibit microorganism growth throughout the product's shelf life and use according to labeling. Refer to Section 3.8, Finished IVD Inspection and Testing, for further discussion.

C) Some IVDs that contain microorganisms cannot be filtered, nor contain microbiological inhibitory systems, because product performance would be adversely affected. Consequently, microorganisms are likely to be present in the product. The allowable level of contamination that will not adversely affect product performance throughout the IVD's shelf life is determined, and appropriate specifications and accept/reject criteria are established to ensure this level is not exceeded at the end of production and during controlled storage. Depending on the specific type of product, specifications usually address batch contamination (percent contamination of a lot through its labeled shelf life) or contamination per unit (slide, plate, etc.). Typically, these microbiologically controlled IVDs are manufactured by designing a manufacturing process which limits the presence of microorganisms; and, by controlling the contamination of product components through sterilization, aseptic technique, or filtration. In addition to limiting the amount of microorganisms present, some IVDs may be capable of having only specific types of microorganisms which would not adversely affect product performance. In this case, the specific types of microorganisms are identified and limited according to the product's established specifications which assure that product function is not adversely affected through its expected shelf life and use according to labeling.

3.2 Process Validation

Section 820.5 requires that every finished device manufacturer prepare and implement a quality assurance program that is appropriate to the specific device manufactured. Section 820.3(n) defines quality assurance as all activities necessary to assure and verify confidence in the quality of the process used to manufacture a finished device. Section 820.100 requires that written manufacturing specifications and processing procedures be established, implemented, and controlled to assure that the device conforms to its original design or any approved changes in that design. Section 820.100(a)(1) requires that procedures for specification control measures be established to assure that the design basis for the device, components, and packaging is correctly translated into approved specifications. These four GMP sections establish the requirements for process validation, as stated in FDA's "Guideline on General Principles of Process Validation."*(2)* It is suggested that this guideline be consulted when establishing validation procedures. The following are a means of meeting process validation requirements.

Process validation is defined as establishing documented evidence which provides a high degree of assurance that a specified process will consistently produce a product meeting its predetermined specifications and quality attributes. The process is validated using accepted methods after defining the manufacturing process, including the equipment, the environment in which the operation is to be performed, and the quality assurance controls to be applied. When validating a process, the interaction of all systems is evaluated. Process validation applies to all three microbiological categories of IVDs to ensure that a specified process will consistently produce an IVD which meets all specifications and quality attributes. Validation may be prospective or retrospective, or a combination of both.

All new IVDs and/or processes are to be prospectively validated. Prospective validation is performed for IVDs which are labeled as sterile because of the limitations of finished product sterility testing. Prospective validation is also used for microbiologically controlled IVDs and for microbiologically uncontrolled IVDs because of the limitations of statistical sampling.

Retrospective validation is the examination and evaluation of historical data for the process and the product. Where retrospective validation is planned for all or part of the manufacturing process for an old product, preproduction process development, qualification, documentation, and process data collection are carefully and appropriately done. Retrospective validation is not used to justify a bad system or a bad product. It is intended to be used to examine a system objectively and determine whether it is acceptable, whether changes need to be made, or whether the entire process needs to be replaced.

In some cases, retrospective validation may be used for IVDs which have been marketed without sufficient premarket process validation. It may be possible to validate, in some measure, the adequacy of the process by examination of accumulated test data and manufacturing records. Retrospective validation encompasses: a review of the process design; determining whether adequate specifications have been established and met for each processing variable; determining whether adequate test methods and sampling plans were established, and adequate sampling and testing was performed to provide a significant data base; and, determining whether adequate procedures are in place. Process and product test data may be useful only if the methods and results are adequate and specific. Specific results can be statistically analyzed and a determination can be made of what variance in data can be expected. Records which describe each process variable are maintained. When test data is used to demonstrate conformance to specifications, the test methodology is qualified to ensure that test results are objective and accurate. Retrospective validation can be used for microbiologically controlled IVDs and for microbiologically uncontrolled IVDs.

3.3 Production and Process Controls

Section 3.2, Process Validation, outlines the GMP sections applicable to process validation (§ 820.100(a)(1)). FDA has interpreted the GMP regulation to require validation of manufacturing processes such as sterilization, lyophilization, filtration, and filling processes. Section 820.100(a)(2) requires that specification changes be subject to controls as stringent as those applied to the original design specifications of the device. Section 820.100(b)(1) requires that where deviations from device specifications could occur as a result of the manufacturing process itself, there shall be written procedures describing any processing controls necessary to assure conformance to specifications. Complying with these GMP sections involves validation and revalidation, and establishing processing controls, for sterilization and microbiological reduction techniques, lyophilization, filtration, and filling processes.

3.3.1   Sterilization and Microbiological Reduction Techniques

Sterilization of product, containers, closures, and the equipment used in production is accomplished by a variety of different methods or processes. These same techniques can be used to reduce the microbial load of microbiologically controlled products. In general, the sterilization and microbial reduction processes used in the production of IVD products are steam, ethylene oxide, radiation, and dry heat, along with appropriate process controls. The CDRH has published responses to common questions regarding sterilization processes(3). These processes are used in manufacturing IVDs which are labeled sterile; sterilizing components for either IVDs which are labeled sterile, or microbiologically controlled IVDs; and, reducing the microbial load for either microbiologically controlled IVDs or microbiologically uncontrolled IVDs.

Saturated steam is used for terminal sterilization or for reducing a microbial load. Guidance for the qualification of autoclaves and validation of autoclave cycles is found in the Parenteral Drug Association (PDA) Technical Monograph No. 1: "Validation of Steam Sterilization Cycles."*(4)*

Ethylene oxide (EO) has some limited uses in IVD manufacturing. The Association for the Advancement of Medical Instrumentation (AAMI) "Guideline for Industrial Ethylene Oxide Sterilization of Medical Devices" contains guidance for the qualification of sterilization chambers and for the validation of EO process cycles*(5)*.

Gamma radiation also has some limited uses in IVD manufacturing and is usually a contracted service. The AAMI "Process Control Guidelines for Gamma Radiation Sterilization of Medical Devices" contains guidance for gamma radiation processes*(6)*.

Dry heat has some limited uses in IVD manufacturing. The PDA Technical Report for "Validation of Dry Heat Processes Used for Sterilization and Depyrogenation" contains guidance for the qualification and validation of dry heat chambers and processes*(7)*.

3.3.2 Lyophilization

Lyophilization may adversely affect the sterility or microorganism load, potency, activity, and stability of the final product if not properly validated and controlled. The lyophilization process is validated as part of overall process validation. The general principles of process validation found in the FDA process validation guideline apply*(2)*. Specific guidance is found in several technical references*(8)(9)*. A basic understanding of the process provides insight into the variables which need to be controlled.

Lyophilization essentially consists of the following: freezing an aqueous product; evacuating the lyophilization chamber, usually below 0.1 torr (100 microns Hg); subliming ice on a cold condensing surface at a temperature below that of the product (the condensing surface is within the chamber or in a connecting chamber or unit); and, introducing heat under controlled conditions to dehydrate the product.

Equipment is qualified to show it is capable of monitoring and controlling lyophilization process parameters such as pressure, vacuum, temperature, and time so that the desired moisture levels in the final product are reproducible. Qualification of the lyophilizer includes calibration of gauges such as thermometers, timers, and recorders, and also includes a "vacuum hold" to test for chamber leaks which could adversely affect the final product.

As stated previously, some IVDs are filtered and then aseptically filled into sterile containers. Because the containers usually remain open during the drying process, air is evacuated, and clean air or inert gas, such as nitrogen, is reintroduced into the chamber during the lyophilization process to prevent contamination. The product is protected from contamination during transfer from the filling area to the lyophilizer, while in the freeze-drying chamber, and at the end of the drying process until the containers are sealed. For sterile and microbiologically controlled IVDs, the exhaust and input ports of the chamber have terminal sterilizing filters so that contaminants do not enter the chamber. The filters are periodically replaced, or periodically sterilized and integrity tested. Similar controls are instituted for other IVDs to ensure that the production process does not introduce contaminants which adversely affect product performance.

The final moisture content of the product is specified. If testing is performed as part of process validation, testing on each manufactured lot would not be required as long as the lot is lyophilized within the validated cycle parameters. Failure to maintain an acceptable moisture content may result in a final product that is subpotent, less active, or less stable than labeled.

Adequate cleaning or disinfection of the chamber's internal surfaces including the water condensate drain lines may be necessary. The drains are not connected to sewer lines without atmospheric breaks or back flow prevention equipment.

3.3.3   Filtration

Filtration is used in IVD manufacturing to remove particulates, to sterilize, and to reduce a microbial load. Filtration is frequently used for sterilization or to reduce a microbial load because some IVDs are heat labile. To prevent the reintroduction of particulates or microorganisms, filtration is usually accompanied by dispensing the filtered component or final product into a clean and/or presterilized container within a controlled environment.

The compatibility between the product and the filter is normally determined during validation of the filtration process. Filters are constructed from a variety of different synthetic materials, and assurance is obtained during the validation process that the substrate and solvents used in IVD production do not react with the filter material. Reactions with the filter material can change the filter porosity allowing contaminants to pass, or denature the filter material adding chemical components to the final product which could adversely affect product performance.

Some filtration operations use either pressure or vacuum to force the product through the filter. Filter manufacturers rate their filters to indicate the maximum pressure or vacuum to be applied to the face of the filter. Some IVDs contain macromolecules such as polypeptides. These viscous products have slower filtration flow rates; therefore, longer filtration times and/or larger membrane areas are required. Appropriate controls are in place to ensure the maximum rating is not exceeded. Filter suitability encompasses the flowing applicable areas: flow rates, throughputs, sterilizability, extractables, particles, product stability, toxicity, compatibility of product, and pyrogenicity.

Guidelines for validating filters have been published, and may be used when assessing the adequacy of filter validation*(10)(11) (12)(13)*. Filter manufacturers may have already validated their filters for bacterial retention. Some of the more complex validation tests are performed by filter manufacturers or contract laboratories, and the test data applying to the IVD manufactured is accessible to the IVD manufacturer.

Because a filter may contain pores larger than the nominal rating, and the probability of microorganism passage increases as the number of organisms in the filtered material increases, a maximum bioburden is established and the filter is challenged using that bioburden. *Pseudomonas diminuta* is normally used for challenging a filter's nominal porosity and for simulating the smallest microorganism occurring in production. Once production begins, product bioburden is controlled, and periodic testing ensures that maximum levels are not exceeded. If bioburden limits are exceeded, an investigation is performed to identify and correct the cause.

Terminal filtration of soluble liquid IVDs for purposes of sterilization or microbial reduction involves the use of a terminal bacterial retentive filter, which has a 0.2 micrometer or smaller pore size rating for most products. Membrane filters are rated by absolute pore size, while depth filters are rated by absolute and nominal pore size. Occasionally, for products with high viscosity or high colloidal content that inhibit filtration through 0.2 micrometer filters, it may be possible to exclude certain microorganisms by using 0.45 micrometer filters in series. Filters of 0.45 micrometer porosity or larger are also useful as pre-filters in extending the life of the terminal filter.

Filtration of some IVDs involves the removal of bacteria, yeasts, and molds. Some IVDs are also filtered to exclude specified interfering mycoplasma, rickettsia, and viruses; however, even a 0.1 micrometer filter may not totally remove these contaminants. If filtration does not remove a contaminant which will adversely affect performance, appropriate and adequate process controls are established to prevent the introduction of the contaminant into the component or finished IVD. In the event the prohibited contaminant is detected, appropriate corrective measures are established.

After validating the filtration process, the manufacturing process, and filter for a given IVD or related class of IVDs, other factors are considered to ensure that replacement filters will perform in the same manner. Procedures are established to ensure that replacement filters are installed in accordance with the filter manufacturer's instructions. The failure to install a filter properly is not necessarily reflected in the ability of the filter to pass a pre-use or post-use integrity test. Filter integrity testing is accomplished as often as necessary to ensure the integrity of the filter and adequacy of the process.

3.3.4   Filling Processes

The following is a discussion of filling processes and their validation for IVDs labeled as sterile, microbiologically controlled IVDs, and microbiologically uncontrolled IVDs.

Aseptic processing may be used to process devices intended to be labeled sterile if the process can achieve a SAL of at least 10^{-3}. An aseptically processed product is likely to consist of components which have been maintained in a sterile condition or have been processed by one of the previously described sterilization processes. USP states that aseptic processing is "...designed to prevent the introduction of viable microorganisms into components, where sterile, or once an intermediate process has rendered the bulk product or its components free from viable microorganisms."*(14)* The container and closure system and applicable production equipment are separately subjected to sterilization processes. Because no further processing occurs after the product is in its final container, production occurs in a controlled environment to maintain product sterility. Manipulation of the product, containers, or closures prior to or during aseptic processing increases the risk of contamination and is controlled as much as possible. Guidance for aseptic processing operations can be found in FDA's "Guideline on Sterile Drug Products Produced by Aseptic Processing."*(15)*

An aseptic processing area or facility for IVDs labeled sterile typically includes some of the following conditions and controls: non-porous, smooth surfaces on floors, walls, and ceilings which can be sanitized or disinfected easily; gowning areas or rooms with adequate space for personnel, garment storage, soiled garment disposal, and hand washing; adequate separation of personnel preparation rooms from the aseptic room by means of airlocks, pass-through windows for components, supplies, and equipment; and, access limited to authorized personnel*(16)(17)*. Training programs and procedures are developed to ensure that all materials brought into the primary environment have been adequately decontaminated or controlled. Specifications for environmentally controlled areas are contained in the device master record.

HEPA filtered enclosures are used particularly in and over the immediate area of the exposed product. Some aseptic processing of IVDs is performed in a HEPA filtered, unidirectional airflow cabinet. Other IVDs which are potentially infective are processed in HEPA filtered biological safety cabinets which are negative in pressure to the secondary environment to protect the worker and the product.

The production and process controls necessary to produce IVDs labeled sterile are well defined in existing guidelines*(15)(18)(19)*. Similar processes used by manufacturers who do not intend to produce sterile devices or IVDs labeled sterile, but are attempting to achieve a certain level of microbiological control, have not been well defined. However, regardless of the process utilized, it is defined in terms of the desired results and allowable operating parameters. These are translated into written process specifications and maintained in the device master record.

A microbiologically controlled IVD is likely to consist of components which have been processed or maintained with a controlled microbial load. The container and closure systems may also be processed to sterile conditions or conditions that will ensure a low microbial load. Because no further processing occurs after the product is in its final container, production is performed in a controlled environment to prevent an increase in the product's microbial load beyond its design specifications.

A microbiologically uncontrolled IVD does not normally have as stringent controls as those for IVDs which are labeled as sterile or for microbiologically controlled IVDs. Appropriate production and process controls are defined in written specifications and instituted to ensure that each filled unit is capable of meeting its established performance specifications. This includes items such as volume of fill, closure integrity, and prevention of contamination during the filling process which adversely affects product performance.

3.3.4.1   Validation of Filling Processes

Aseptic processes are validated because finished product testing for sterility or contamination has limited usefulness. USP, Section 1211, Aseptic Processing states "Certification and validation of the aseptic process and facility is achieved by establishing the efficiency of the filtration systems, by employing microbiological environmental monitoring procedures, and by processing of sterile culture medium as simulated product. Monitoring of the aseptic facility should include periodic environmental filter examination as well as routine particulate and microbiological environmental monitoring, and may include periodic sterile culture medium processing."*(14)*

Guidance for the validation of liquid IVD aseptic fill operations is found in PDA Technical Monograph No. 2, "Validation of Aseptic Filling for Solution Drug Products."*(18)* Guidance for the validation of dry IVD aseptic fill operations is found in PDA Technical Monograph No. 6, "Validation of Aseptic Drug Powder Filling Processes."*(19)* FDA's "Guideline on Sterile Drug Products by Aseptic Processing" provides detailed guidance on validation by media fills*(15)*. Fill processes used to produce sterile IVDs are validated to a SAL of at least 10^{-3}*(18)*. A sufficient number of containers are filled that will provide a high degree of probability of detecting contaminated units. For example, on a statistical basis, using the formula $P(x>0) = 1-e^{-NP}>0.95$, at least 3,000 units are needed to detect a contamination rate of one in one thousand units (0.1%) with a high degree of probability (95% confidence)*(18)*.

Some aseptically filled IVDs consist of lot sizes smaller than 3,000 units. For these smaller lot sizes, each validation run consists of the maximum lot size produced. However, more than three runs are necessary to achieve a high degree of probability (95% confidence) of detecting a contamination rate of 0.1%. Statistically equivalent rationale is developed for other lot sizes, using the formula for a 95% probability or greater for detecting at least one contaminated unit.

The prospective validation procedures for producing microbiologically controlled IVDs closely parallels the same procedures used for IVDs which are labeled sterile. Validation assures that the intended microbiological assurance level (MAL), or other specification for microbial contamination, is achieved consistently. Unlike validation of an aseptic filling process which is used to produce sterile products, validation of microbiologically controlled filling processes is intended to ensure that each filled unit is within established specifications for microorganism levels.

The prospective validation procedures for producing microbiologically uncontrolled IVDs are not as complex as those for IVDs which are labeled as sterile or for microbiologically controlled IVDs. Rather than determining contamination levels, the operation is validated to ensure that it is capable of filling each unit within a run to meet its established performance specifications. This includes such items as volume of fill, closure integrity, and prevention of contamination during the filling process which adversely affects product performance. Of course, these items are also a concern with microbiologically controlled IVDs and IVDs which are labeled sterile.

Each filling line or filling operation is validated, and sufficient validation runs are performed to ensure results are statistically meaningful and consistent. Usually three separate runs are recognized by industry as adequate(20). The number of validation runs is dependent on the need to demonstrate repeatability of the filling process.

Since sampling plans for finished product testing normally carry some inherent risk of allowing defective lots to be accepted, filling processes are revalidated at predetermined intervals or as necessary to ensure that all processes, procedures, and training programs are still adequate. Some additional reasons for revalidation include: building and equipment changes, personnel changes, environmental specifications being exceeded, positive sterility or microbial limits test results, and the failure of IVD lots to meet specifications. Because of the limits of finished product testing, periodic revalidation is performed even in the absence of apparent changes.

Microbiological media, rather than actual product, is normally used to validate a filling process where the intent is to produce a sterile product or to limit microbial contamination. The media for validation runs is chosen for its capability of supporting the growth of microorganisms previously identified by environmental monitoring and by positive sterility tests. Negative and positive controls are used to ensure the validity of the runs. The growth medium and growth promotion organisms listed in USP are generally acceptable for media validation runs. The filled media units from each run are incubated at a sufficient temperature and time period to detect microorganisms. For product labeled as sterile, this would be 7 or 14 days incubation, depending on the sterility test method employed, and it would be 3 days for microbial limits testing. Where more than one medium or incubation condition is used to detect all potential contaminants, failure or contamination rates are calculated separately for each type of medium utilized during validation, and separate failure or contamination rates are calculated within each medium type when incubated at separate temperatures.

The production environment during filling process validation is challenged at the upper process limits. Some of the items to consider are the number of personnel present in the area, activity levels, temperature, humidity, pressure differentials, and other environmental factors. The duration of each validation and revalidation run encompasses most, if not all, processing steps during actual production operations.

In cases where adequate prospective validation has not been performed for old microbiologically controlled IVDs or old microbiologically uncontrolled IVDs, retrospective validation may be appropriate. Product test data, complaint file analysis, trend analysis, bioburden studies, and process control data, along with an examination of the buildings, equipment, employee technique, and clothing requirements, may be capable of showing whether the presence of microorganisms in the IVD can or cannot adversely affect product performance. A limited prospective validation may be necessary to verify the retrospective study results, especially if inadequate historical data has been collected.

3.4 Environmental Control

Section 820.46 requires that where environmental conditions at the manufacturing site could have an adverse effect on the fitness for use of a device, these environmental conditions must be controlled to prevent contamination of the device and to provide proper conditions for each of the operations performed pursuant to

Section 820.40. This section states that any environmental control system must be periodically inspected to verify that the system is properly functioning, and such inspections must be documented.

Conditions to be considered for control include: lighting, ventilation, temperature, humidity, air pressure, filtration, airborne contamination, and other contamination. Guidance regarding environmental control is found and referenced in Federal Standard 209D "Clean Room and Work Station Requirements, Controlled Environment."*(21)* The controls needed depend on the type of IVD being produced, and is usually determined, in part, by the product specifications. The following environmental controls apply chiefly to IVDs which are labeled sterile and microbiologically controlled IVDs, but could also apply to microbiologically uncontrolled IVDs. The following are means of complying with the GMP requirements for establishing environmental controls and environmental monitoring for airborne contamination, air pressure, and filtration.

3.4.1   Airborne and Other Contamination

Non-viable particle monitoring is a fast method for indicating area particle contamination levels and is done during validation of the filling process and on a scheduled basis during production. Monitoring is performed at several locations throughout the product exposure period under dynamic conditions.

Reasonable and feasible specifications for non-viable particles are established for controlled environment processing areas. The specifications are verified during process validation as being adequate, and alert and action levels are established. Non-viable particle specifications are established for processing in unidirectional airflow hoods. Because of the possibility of the transfer of contaminants by equipment and employees, particle specifications are also established for the room in which the hood is located. Specifications are established for biological safety cabinets and for the room in which the cabinet is located. Specifications account for the fact that biological safety cabinets utilize room air to create a negative pressure in the hood and a positive pressure in the room.

Viable particle monitoring is performed during process validation and on a scheduled basis during production. Active air samplers are used to quantify the number of microorganisms present in an area. Active samplers include slit-to-agar samplers, sieve samplers, liquid impingement samplers, and centrifugal agar samplers. Passive air samplers, such as settling plates, have limited value in quantitative monitoring, particularly under unidirectional airflow, because microorganisms that do not settle onto plates are not detected. However, they can be valuable in qualitative monitoring: 1) if positioned in critical areas; 2) if they can effectively capture microorganisms; and, 3) if exposure is not so prolonged as to dry the nutrient*(22)*. Environmental monitoring to be considered also includes: touch plate, contact plate, and swab testing of critical surfaces such as floors, walls, ceilings, equipment, utensils, and personnel clothing.

Viable particle monitoring methods, in order to be effective, are shown to be capable of detecting all contaminants of concern. The microbiological culture media used in viable monitoring is incubated at appropriate times, temperatures, and environmental conditions. Any recovered microorganisms are identified to differentiate between normal and incidental contaminants. Although every isolate need not be identified to genus and species, characterization is specific enough: 1) to establish a data base that will demonstrate that cleaning and disinfecting continue to be effective; 2) to establish a relationship between organisms found during prospective validation and finished product testing; and, 3) to determine the resistance of environmental organisms to various sterilization or contamination control processes.

Reasonable and feasible specifications for viable particles are established for controlled environment processing areas. The specifications are verified during process validation as being adequate, and alert and action levels are established. The various processing areas are evaluated, with more stringent limits set in those areas where the product is exposed to the environment, or primary environment, versus secondary environments.

3.4.2   Air Pressure

Air pressure differential specifications are established between primary controlled areas and secondary controlled areas. Quantitatively measurable pressure differential monitoring between the primary controlled areas and secondary controlled areas is performed, and conformance to established specifications is verified. The adequacy of the specifications are verified during process validation, and alert and action levels are established. Controlled environment areas have a positive pressure in relation to areas of lesser control. However, for biological safety cabinets or rooms designed for containment of infectious agents, the primary environment has a negative pressure with respect to the surrounding environment*(23)*.

3.4.3 Filtration

Air filtration is commonly used to help maintain environmental control in a processing area. Reasonable and feasible specifications for non-viable particles are established for controlled environment processing areas. The adequacy of the air filtration system, and the specifications for the system, are verified during process validation.

When controlled environmental conditions are being maintained through the use of HEPA filters, the HEPA filters are certified to be 99.97% efficient in the retention of particles 0.3 micrometer or larger. This is usually done via a DOP test. A certificate of DOP conformance is usually supplied by the filter manufacturer; if not, the IVD manufacturer certifies conformance. Upon installation of the filter and again periodically thereafter (e.g., twice a year), the HEPA filters are integrity tested by the DOP test or equivalent test methods. Whether the frequency of periodic testing is increased or decreased is dependent on the data obtained from previous testing. Periodic quantitative monitoring is performed to ensure HEPA filters are operating within specifications. HEPA filters can enclose entire rooms, can be in a work station, or can be in a unidirectional airflow work station.

In addition to HEPA filters, terminal air filters, used in other controlled environment areas of the firm, are tested upon receipt, or accepted by certificate of conformance, to ensure their retentive capabilities in order to meet the air quality specifications for those areas. Periodic quantitative monitoring is performed to ensure terminal filters are operating within specifications.

Work stations used in the production of infectious agents are certified periodically (e.g., annually) to meet the standards for Type II or Type III Biological Safety Cabinets*(23)*. These certifications establish the filter efficiency and also test the cabinet for leaks that would compromise containment requirements.

3.5 Personnel Attire

Section 820.56(a) requires that where special clothing requirements are necessary to ensure that a device is fit for its intended use, clean dressing rooms are provided. Section 820.25(b) requires that personnel in contact with a device or its environment are clean, healthy, and suitably attired where lack of cleanliness, good health, or suitable attire could adversely affect the device. The following are a means of complying with these GMP sections for determining and establishing personnel attire requirements.

The extent to which clothing procedures and practices are established, validated, and controlled are based on the type of IVD being produced, and are usually determined, in part, by the product specifications.

Where the primary processing environment for IVDs is a controlled environment room or area, appropriate clothing is used to ensure product and process specifications are met. These may include the following items, when appropriate: coveralls, open-face or eyes-only hood, surgical face mask, shoe covers or boots, and surgical gloves. When primary processing is limited to a unidirectional airflow hood or biological safety cabinet, located in a secondary environment, less stringent clothing practices may be employed, such as full-cover lab coat, hair restraint, surgical face mask (if no face shield is present on the hood), and sterile sleeves, and/or gloves.

When aseptic processing is used, proper aseptic gowning practices are essential. Aseptic gowning practices include sterile gloves for handling sterile garments. At the conclusion of the gowning process, these gloves are removed and new sterile gloves put on, or the old gloves are thoroughly cleaned and disinfected. During the gowning procedure, caution is followed to protect sterile garments from contacting non-sterile surfaces which may contaminate the garments. As people generate particles during activity, sleeves and pant legs of the sterile garments are tucked inside the gloves and boot/shoe covers to prevent particles from flushing out of the gown into the environment. Once removed, sterile clothing is not normally reused to enter aseptic areas, unless the practice is validated. Once an employee has moved from a controlled environment to a non-controlled environment, the employee does not re-enter the aseptic area without regowning, unless the process is validated to show that the employee does not add unacceptable contaminants to the aseptic area.

The use of sterile clothing is the most reliable means of assuring that clothing does not contribute contamination. If sterile clothing is not used, the acceptability of non-sterile clothing is determined during validation. Verification of the effectiveness of all clothing procedures and practices for controlled environment operations is part of validation. Validation includes contact sampling at several sites on each individual immediately after gowning to establish baseline data. Alert and action limits for contamination are established above which it is reasonably expected that an employee is compromising the controlled environment. If this occurs, employee retraining and/or removal from the controlled environment are alternative actions. Employee gowning practices are periodically monitored as part of an ongoing quality assurance program.

3.6 Cleaning and Sanitation

Section 820.56 requires adequate written cleaning procedures and schedules to meet manufacturing process specifications, and that such procedures are provided to appropriate personnel. The following are means of complying with this GMP section for determining and establishing cleaning and sanitation requirements.

The effectiveness of the cleaning process is determined as part of process validation. Cleaning and disinfecting agents used to clean equipment, floors, and walls need to be effective against the microorganisms which may adversely affect product function. The effectiveness of the cleaning process is verified and documented using swabs or contact plates as part of validation. Once validated, the cleaning process is monitored but may use fewer sampling sites than used during validation. This monitoring may be performed as part of an overall environmental monitoring program.

Acceptable monitoring results would indicate either no viable microorganisms present, or a reduced bioburden which has been demonstrated by process validation to not adversely affect the final product. When results show that the established limits have been exceeded, an investigation is performed to identify the source of the contamination. The cleaning process is repeated as necessary.

Cleaning equipment is stored in a dedicated, controlled area in order to protect the controlled environment area and its equipment from contamination. Water used to prepare cleaning and disinfectant solutions for controlled areas will have low microorganism levels.

3.7 Components

GMP requirements for components are stated in § 820.20(a)(2) and § 820.80. Section 820.181(a) requires that the device master record include or refer to the location of component specifications. All raw materials, containers, and closures are considered components. Packaging requirements for IVD containers and closures stated in § 820.181(d) and § 820.130 also apply. The following are several means of complying with these GMP sections for components.

Where deviations from component specifications could result in the device being unfit for its intended use, components are inspected, sampled, and tested for conformance to specifications, or certificates of analysis are obtained from the supplier in lieu of testing upon receipt. Confidence in the validity of certificates is established through experience, historical data, testing, and audits of the supplier. If the device master record contains specifications in addition to those listed in the supplier's certification, then the IVD manufacturer ascertains that the component meets these additional specifications. For those components where a supplier does not perform any testing, or components are manufactured in-house, the IVD manufacturer ascertains that adequate specifications are established and appropriate examinations or tests, as necessary, are performed to ensure these specifications are met. For those components which are intended to be sterile or have a low microorganism load to ensure IVD specifications are met, acceptable levels of bacteria, yeasts, molds, viruses, rickettsia, and mycoplasma, as appropriate, are addressed through established specifications which are then monitored. If any detectable level of endotoxins in the final product would adversely affect product performance, the susceptible components are tested for the presence of endotoxins.

Water is used for a variety of purposes, such as in sterilization systems, preparation of cleaning agents, and in product formulations. Water used in the production of IVDs is as important as any other product component. Water quality is defined as any other product component, and the specifications are consistent with the performance characteristics of the final product. Specifications are established for water used in the product and processing. The equipment used to produce the water is qualified and certified. The system is validated to ensure it produces the quality of water it is intended to produce, and the system is routinely monitored to ensure that the quality of the water continues to meet the established specifications. Water for IVD production purposes is usually produced by deionization, distillation, and/or reverse osmosis.

Water used in production may not need to be sterile, except when added aseptically to a sterile product. If the microbial load present in the process water could adversely affect the finished product, then microbiological specification limits are established for the water. An increase in bioburden of water and/or other components may adversely affect the ability of a sterilization process to effectively sterilize a product, or keep a microbiologically controlled IVD within acceptable limits. Thus, monitoring of the microbial load in water is important.

Some IVDs are chemically defined. Therefore, establishing specifications and controlling and testing the ionic and chemical quality of the process water are important in limiting impurities which could adversely affect the IVD.

If detectable levels of endotoxin in the final IVD can adversely affect performance, then it may be necessary to limit gram negative bacteria in the water, establish endotoxin limits, and test the water for endotoxins. Water used in some IVDs may need to have low levels or be free of endotoxins*(24)*. Maximum allowable endotoxin specifications are established from validation data which shows that product performance would not be adversely affected by the permissible limits established.

Points of control for process water systems used in manufacturing IVDs include: 1) proper temperature maintenance in the storage tank; 2) pressure gauges and pressure specifications at various points throughout the system; 3) the absence of dead legs; 4) the absence of in-line bacterial retentive filters (to prevent bacterial build-up on the upstream side, resulting in pyrogen release and bacterial breakthrough) unless their use can be properly validated and monitored; and, 5) the absence of direct sewer connections to the water system, including such situations as hoses attached to water outlets that extend below the top level of sinks, or that contact floors or other non-sanitized surfaces unless they are removed after use. A disinfection and/or sterilization procedure and schedule is established for the entire water system, as necessary, to ensure bioburden specifications are maintained.

3.8 Finished IVD Inspection and Testing

Section 820.20(a)(2) requires that the quality assurance program consist of procedures adequate to ensure proper approval or rejection of all finished devices, and approval or rejection of devices manufactured, processed, packaged, or held under contract by another company. Section 820.20(a)(4) requires that the quality assurance program consist of procedures to ensure that all quality assurance checks are appropriate and adequate for their purpose and are performed correctly. Section 820.160 requires written procedures for finished device inspections to ensure that device specifications are met. The following are means of complying with these GMP sections for finished IVD inspection and testing.

In addition to process validation and in-process controls, adequate sampling and testing of the finished product helps to confirm that manufacturing processes were correctly performed, and that the product will consistently accomplish its intended function within labeled claims, such as accuracy, precision, sensitivity, specificity, sterility, purity, and identity.

Section 820.160 requires that sampling plans for checking, testing, and release of a device be based on an acceptable statistical rationale. Sampling programs are designed and implemented by each manufacturer. They include the establishment of an Acceptable Quality Level (AQL) and selection of a sampling plan that provides an acceptable level of confidence that defective lots, such as those in which the defect rate exceeds the AQL, will be detected and rejected.

There are no simple rules for selecting a value for the AQL, but it is usually product specific and is based on the rate of defects which can be tolerated both by the user and the manufacturer for the specific indicated uses of the IVD. If the IVD has multiple uses, prudence indicates that the value, consistent with the process capability, which produces the best protection for the most sensitive use be selected. Once the AQL is selected, a quality control sampling plan is selected and implemented which will provide an acceptable level of confidence that lots in which the defect rate exceeds the AQL have a suitably high probability of detection and rejection. These plans are based on accepted statistical principles, and documentation is available to support the statistical validity of the plan.

When the selection of the sampling plan is complete, the risks involved in applying the plan need to be understood. This includes such factors as the probability of accepting a lot whose quality is as good or better than the AQL and the risk of accepting a lot with a defect rate which exceeds the AQL. An acceptable plan provides a high degree of confidence commensurate with the significance of the use of the device and the needs of the user. Any sampling plan is valid only if the manufacturing operation is in a complete state of control, as determined through process capability studies or validation.

The sampling plan in use also assures that the samples are representative of the lot. Samples obtained from a filling operation are representative of the lot if they are obtained periodically throughout the filling run, and include the beginning, middle, and end of the filling run. If retesting of the lot is performed, because the initial testing found that the lot failed to meet one or more of its specifications, then the sampling plan being used for the retest accounts for a tightened inspection plan by obtaining a larger number of samples.

Section 820.160 requires that finished devices be held in quarantine or otherwise adequately controlled until released. In most cases, finished IVDs are adequately controlled to prevent release until testing is completed and the products are approved for distribution. FDA allows release of certain finished IVDs before testing is complete if they have a short shelf life, and the length of time required for completion of testing would equal or exceed the IVDs' expiration date. However, if it is found that specifications have not been met upon completion of finished product testing, appropriate corrective action, such as a recall, may be necessary.

Section 820.160 requires that prior to release for distribution, each production run, lot, or batch is checked and, where necessary, tested for conformance with device specifications. It also requires that, where practical, a device shall be selected from a production run, lot, or batch and tested under simulated use conditions. The following are several types of common tests performed on IVDs and suggested ways of complying with this section of the GMP regulation.

Finished product testing generally involves testing a reagent and associated items, or all reagents which are part of a diagnostic system, such as an IVD kit, together to confirm they will function properly as a system. Validated test methods, calibrated equipment, and appropriate traceable standards used in testing are specified to the customer in the product's labeling. Testing assures that each lot is capable of performing accurately with each instrument recommended to the user in the product's labeling. Each lot may not need to be tested on each instrument specified to the user. For example, some of the tests on certain specified instruments can be performed during the product design phase.

Sometimes, it is not possible for a manufacturer to interchange reagents among kits from different lots without adversely affecting performance. If kit reagents are interchanged, the "new" finished device kit may require reevaluation to determine whether it meets labeled performance specifications. If replacing IVD kit reagents with reagents from a different lot can adversely affect product performance, the user is warned of potential problems via labels and other labeling.

The identity of each production lot is verified to ensure compliance with its labeling. Identity tests are performed where visual or other routine inspection or testing alone is insufficient to determine identity. Identity tests in use will depend on the specific product and its labeling claims. Appropriate identity tests that consider the preceding points are designed to distinguish the specific product from any other similar product. In some cases, adequate process validation along with adequate process control may be satisfactory in lieu of identity testing.

Turbidity in a product may not establish that a product is contaminated; however, it may indicate the necessity of investigating the cause, and may be a reason for rejection. The clarity of fluids is not an acceptable proof of sterility because contaminating microorganisms may not always result in turbidity. Further, some products are characteristically turbid; in which case, turbidity would not be a basis for rejection.

Media used to test the final product for sterility testing or microbial limits testing are comparable to those identified in the USP, and are performance tested prior to use in accordance with USP*(14)*. If an IVD contains antibiotics or preservatives, which could mask the presence of microorganisms, the antibiotics or preservatives are inactivated prior to testing in order to detect the potential contaminants.

Some IVDs are their own growth media. Incubation of the finished IVD samples under appropriate conditions and temperatures is performed to detect a wide range of microorganisms. Of course, the finished IVD is also tested to ensure that it supports or inhibits the growth of microorganisms, or exhibits the expected reaction for which it was formulated.

Microbiological inhibitory systems such as antibiotics, preservatives, pH control, or antisera are added to some IVDs to inhibit microbial contamination. The USP states that antimicrobial preservatives "... are used primarily in multiple-dose containers to inhibit the growth of microorganisms that may be introduced inadvertently, during or subsequent to, the manufacturing process. Antimicrobial agents should not be used solely to reduce the viable microbial count as a substitute for good manufacturing practice."*(14)* While this section in the USP speaks of drug dosage forms, the information is applicable to IVDs. Microbiological inhibitory systems are used for some sterile IVDs to prevent contamination during distribution, storage, or multiple entries into the container by the user. Microbiological inhibitory systems are used in microbiologically controlled IVDs to keep the microbial load at an acceptable level, and to ensure that multiple entry by the customer does not allow the proliferation of microorganisms which could make the product unfit for its intended use. Also, the remains or byproducts of microorganisms may adversely affect product performance. Microbiological inhibitory systems are set at inhibitory levels that will control contamination and yet not adversely affect product performance, and this is determined during preproduction product development and pilot production. Assurance that the microbial levels present in the IVD do not exceed the capability of the microbiological inhibitory system is provided by process validation and periodic product monitoring for microbial limits. Preservative effectiveness levels may be tested using appropriate methods, such as USP, Section 51*(14)*. Other types of microbiological inhibitory systems can be tested using appropriate validated test methods.

3.9 *Stability Studies and Expiration Testing*

Section 820.100(a)(1) requires that procedures for specification control measures be established to ensure that the design basis for the device, components, and packaging is correctly translated into approved specifications. When IVD stability is a design concern, appropriate procedures such as stability studies are conducted and an expiration period, supported by the studies, is established to define the period in which stability is assured. The expiration period is included as part of the product specifications for the IVD and its components, as required by § 820.181(a).

Stability studies for all IVDs are required by Sections 809.10 (a)(5) and 809.10(b)(5)(iv). These regulations require that storage instructions be stated on the immediate container label, kit, or outer container label. Storage instructions are required in the product insert for the product in its initial state and for products which are mixed or reconstituted prior to use. Where applicable, storage instructions should include temperature, light, and humidity or other conditions. The immediate container label, and the kit or outer container label, are required by § 809.10(a)(6) to state a means by which the user is assured the IVD meets appropriate standards of identity, strength, quality, and purity at time of use. This assurance can be an expiration date, an observable indication of product alteration, such as turbidity, or instructions for a simple function test. The following are means of complying with these regulations for establishing stability studies and expiration dating.

An expiration date is the usual method used to indicate stability for IVDs. The last date for the product to be used by the customer is defined as the expiration date.

The storage instructions and the expiration period are determined as part of product development for the proposed container/closure system. The device package and shipping container are evaluated as part of this development phase. For example, during product development an IVD labeled for storage at 2° to 8°C was found to be stable for 24 months. Studies were performed by the manufacturer which subjected the IVD to adverse shipping temperatures of -5°C and 37°C for one week each; however, the IVD was stable for only 6 months at 2° to 8°C after being subjected to these adverse shipping conditions. A shipping container was then designed to maintain the IVD product at 2° to 8°C during adverse environmental conditions that might be encountered during shipping to support the 24 month expiration period. This type of design effort supports the type of adequate package design requirements of § 820.130.

Storage instructions for IVDs are required by § 809.10(a)(5) to include reliable, meaningful, and specific test methods such as those in §21 CFR 211.166. Section 211.166 requires sample sizes and test intervals to be based on statistical criteria for each attribute examined to ensure valid estimates of stability and also requires reliable, meaningful, and specific test methods. Performance and identity testing on all IVD reagents and systems is included in the stability testing program. In addition, sterility testing on sterile labeled IVDs, and microbial limits testing on all microbiologically controlled IVDs, is included in the stability testing program. The finished IVD product is held under appropriate conditions to support the expiration period and storage instructions determined during the development phase. These are normally taken from the first three production batches.

Currently, FDA accepts only real time data for supporting an expiration period. The sole exception is free-standing liquid controls which are not part of a kit, but an adjunctive and independent control for another diagnostic kit. If real time data is insufficient to support the full expiration period claimed, FDA may, on a case-by-case basis accept accelerated data with the understanding that the data will be supported by real time data, or the shelf life adjusted to reflect the real time expiry.

Each IVD is evaluated for additional stability studies if there is any significant change which may affect stability in the manufacturing process or equipment; in the components, including the container/closure system; or, in the shipping container.

3.10 Complaints and Failure Investigations

Adequate complaint handling systems are required by § 820.198. The following are means of complying with these regulations for maintaining complaints, performing complaint investigations, and performing failure investigations.

A complaint is either a written or oral communication relative to an IVD's identity, quality, durability, reliability, safety, effectiveness, or performance. A written or oral communication which meets the definition of a complaint must be reviewed, evaluated, and maintained by a formally designated unit. The formally designated unit may be an individual or a designated department. If the formally designated unit decides that the complaint does not need to be investigated, a record must be maintained which includes the reason the complaint was not investigated and the name of the individual who made that decision.

A complaint involving the possible failure of an IVD to meet any of its performance specifications must be reviewed, evaluated, and investigated, as required by § 820.198(b). The complainant need only indicate the possible, not confirmed, failure of an IVD.

There are several different mechanisms for receiving complaints. Replacement of a complainant's product has, in many instances, been the basis for deciding not to investigate a complaint any further. This is not an acceptable followup to a report of contaminated product or failure of the IVD to perform within its specifications. If the replacement was performed and it meets the definition of a complaint as defined in § 820.198(a), then the complaint must be reviewed, evaluated, and maintained by a formally designated unit; and, if the complaint involves the possible failure of an IVD to meet any of its performance specifications, then the complaint must be reviewed, evaluated, and investigated. Product credit sheets are routinely maintained by customers which list defective lots, or defective portions of lots, and these sheets are then returned to the IVD manufacturer for credit or replacement of the items. The credit or replacement sheets are reviewed by the formally designated unit to determine which credits or replacements meet the definition of a complaint as defined in § 820.198(a). All credits or replacements which meet the definition of a complaint must be reviewed, evaluated, and maintained; and, if the credit or replacement meets the definition of a complaint, and the complaint involves the possible failure of an IVD to meet any of its performance specifications, then the complaint must be reviewed, evaluated, and investigated. Also, IVD manufacturers routinely manufacture IVDs for themselves and for their own label distributors, other IVD manufacturers, or foreign subsidiaries or manufacturers. The IVD manufacturer has a feedback mechanism in place whereby complaints on their products, received by other organizations, are forwarded to the original manufacturer for review and evaluation.

The extent of a complaint investigation may involve several areas: 1) requesting that the complainant return the product to the manufacturer for examination and testing; 2) examination and testing of the same lot of IVD from the manufacturer's warehouse or reserve sample stock; and, 3) examination of the device history record for the lot to determine if manufacturing and testing procedures were accurately followed, and if all specifications were met prior to release of the IVD lot.

Once the actual failure of a product to meet specifications is identified, the failure investigation requirements of § 820.162 take effect. A written record of the investigation, including conclusions and followup, is required.

If the investigation finds that the lot, or lots, of the IVD do not meet specifications, appropriate corrective action must be instituted. This may include: review of processes and procedures, and making changes where necessary; review of package design and stability studies, and making changes where necessary; and, appropriate corrective action on the remainder of the IVD product in the marketplace, such as recall.

Any complaint pertaining to injury or death, or any hazard to safety, must be immediately reviewed and investigated by a designated individual, and maintained in a separate portion of the complaint file. In addition, complaints must be evaluated to determine if any meet the definition of, and reporting requirements of, medical device reporting as defined in Part 803 of the regulations.

Establishing a written complaint handling procedure is a good quality assurance practice to outline all steps involved in receiving, handling, reviewing, maintaining, and investigating complaints, so that all individuals involved in all aspects of the complaint process are operating under similar directions.

3.11 Trend Analysis

In the July 1978 preamble to the GMP regulation, "statistical control" in proposed § 820.100(c), regarding ongoing trend analysis, was believed to be confusing and essentially duplicating the requirement in § 820.100(b), and was deleted. Section 820.100(b) requires written procedures describing any processing controls necessary to ensure conformance to specifications where deviations from device specifications could occur as a result of the manufacturing process itself. Section 820.20(a)(3) requires that the quality assurance program consist of procedures to identify, recommend, or provide solutions for quality assurance problems and verify the implementation of such solutions. The following are means of complying with these requirements.

Product and process accept/reject data results, along with information from complaint files collected through various documented process and control systems, are evaluated by appropriate methods (e.g., trend analysis) to determine if there are recurring problems or process drift which warrant corrective action. Trend analysis is an important part of an effective quality assurance program and is important for identifying conditions or situations such as performance problems with specific lots or products, seasonal increases in contamination, component vendor problems, or process drift, which might otherwise not be apparent or dismissed as isolated incidents. When such trends are examined, areas of concern or system/process failures may be identified. Measures can then be established and implemented to control or eliminate their reoccurrence.

Appendix I—References

1   Guideline document jointly authored and presented to CDRH by Health Industry Manufacturers Association (HIMA) and Association of Microbiological Diagnostic Manufacturers (AMDM), *Microbial Load Considerations for Prepared Culture Media Products,* HIMA Report No.: IVD 88.13, July 1988, HIMA, Washington, DC 20005.

2   Center for Drugs and Biologics (CDB), and Center for Devices and Radiological Health (CDRH), *Guideline on General Principles of Process Validation, May* 1987, FDA, Division of Manufacturing and Product Quality, HFD-320, 5600 Fishers Lane, Rockville, MD 20857.

3   Manufacturing Quality Assurance Branch, OCS, CDRH, *Sterilization: Questions and Answers from FDA,* April 15, 1985, FDA, HFZ-332, 1390 Piccard Drive, Rockville, MD 20850.

4   *Validation of Steam Sterilization Cycles,* 1978, Parenteral Drug Association (PDA), Philadelphia, PA 19107.

5   *Guideline for Industrial Ethylene Oxide Sterilization of Medical Devices,* March 1988, Association for the Advancement of Medical Instrumentation (AAMI), Arlington, VA 22209.

6   *Process Control Guidelines for Gamma Radiation Sterilization of Medical Devices,* March 1984, AAMI, Arlington, VA 22209.

7   *Validation of Dry Heat Processes Used for Sterilization and Depyrogenation,* 1981, PDA, Philadelphia, PA 19107.

8   T. A. Jennings, *Validation of the Lyophilization Process,* Validation of Aseptic Pharmaceutical Processes, pp 595–633, F.J. Carlton and J.P. Agalloco, ED., 1986.

9   E.H. Trappler and J.Y. Lee, *Validation of Lyophilization,* PDA Annual Meeting, November 16, 1987, PDA, Philadelphia, PA 19107.

10 *Microbiological Evaluation of Filters for Sterilizing Liquids,* Document No. 3, Vol. 4, April 1982, HIMA, Washington, DC 20005.

11 *Validation of Sterilizing Filters,* paper presented in Sweden, May 4, 1981, Millipore Corporation.

12 *Standard Test Method for Determining Bacterial Retention of Membrane Filters Utilized for Liquid Filtration,* American Society for Testing and Material (ASTM), F838-83, ASTM, Philadelphia, PA 19163.

13 *Validation Guide,* Publication TR-680, September 1980, Pall Corp.

14 *The United States Pharmacopeia (USP) and The National Formulary (NF),* The United States Pharmacopeial Convention, Inc., Rockville, MD 20852.

15 *Guideline on Sterile Drug Products Produced by Aseptic Processing,* June 1987, Maintained by FDA, Division of Drug Quality Compliance, HFN-320, 5600 Fishers Lane, Rockville, MD 20857.

16 *Device Good Manufacturing Practices Manual,* 5th Edition, August 1991, FDA, CDRH, HFZ-220, 5600 Fishers Lane, Rockville, MD 20857.

17 *Sterile Medical Devices: A GMP Workshop Manual,* 4th Edition, January 1985, FDA, CDRH, HFZ-220, 5600 Fishers Lane, Rockville, MD 20857.

18 *Validation of Aseptic Filling for Solution Drug Products,* Technical Monograph No. 2, 1980, PDA, Philadelphia, PA 19107.

19 *Validation of Aseptic Drug Powder Filling Processes,* Technical Report No. 6, 1984, PDA, Philadelphia, PA 19107.

20 *HIMA Medical Device Sterilization Monographs: Validation of Sterilization Systems,* Report No.: 78-4.1, June 1978, Health Industries Manufacturers Association (HIMA), Washington, DC 20005.

21 *Federal Standard 209D: Clean Room and Work Station Requirements, Controlled Environment,* June 15, 1988, General Services Administration, Federal Supply Service, Washington, DC 20407.

22 D.B. Detmore & W.N. Thompson, A *Comparison of Air Sampler Efficiencies,* 3:45–48, 52, 1981, Medical Device Diagnostic Industry (MD&DI), Santa Monica, CA 90405.

23 CDC/NIH, *Biosafety in Microbiological and Biomedical Laboratories,* 1st Edition, March 1984, Centers for Disease Control and National Institutes of Health.

24 M.C. Gould, *Endotoxin Vertebrate Cell Culture,* In Vitro Monograph No. 5, page 125, Tissue Culture Association, Gaithersburg, MD 20879.

The following references are also recommended for assuring compliance with the GMP regulation.

25 *FDA Compliance Program Guidance Manual,* Compliance Program (CP) 7382.830, Inspection of Medical Device Manufacturers, October 1988, FDA.

26 *FDA Compliance Program Guidance Manual,* Compliance Program 7382.830A, Sterilization of Medical Devices, October 1988, FDA.

Appendix II—Definitions

Biological Safety Cabinets   primary containment devices in which work may be performed on infectious agents.

Class 100   a clean room or clean zone where the measured particles per cubic foot of size are equal to or greater than any one or more of the following particle sizes: 100 particles per cubic foot of a size 0.5 micrometers and larger; 300 particles per cubic foot of a size 0.3 micrometers and larger; and, 750 particles per cubic foot of a size 0.2 micrometers and larger.

Dead Leg   any section of pipe or other conduit, whose length is six or more times greater than its internal diameter, which is in a fluid distribution system that either carries the fluid through the system or is not drained daily.

Filtered   IVDs which have been processed through a filter greater than 0.22 micrometer in size to remove only certain types of organisms, and their production specifications and product labeling state: 1) the final filter pore size used; 2) the specific viable microorganisms that have and have not been removed from the product by filtration; and, 3) the specific microorganisms whose presence and absence has been confirmed through testing of the finished IVD.

Media Fills   a method of prospectively validating sterile and microbiologically controlled IVD assembly processes using a sterile growth nutrient medium to simulate product filling operations. The nutrient medium is manipulated and exposed to the operators, equipment, containers, closures, surfaces, and environmental conditions to closely simulate the same exposure which the product itself will undergo. The media filled containers are then incubated to determine contamination or whether microbial specifications are met.

Microbiological Assurance Level (MAL)	process specification which assures that microbiologically controlled IVDs are manufactured under appropriate conditions and controls which will result in a product which consistently meets all its specifications, where the MAL is commensurate with the need for safe and effective performance of the IVD.
Microbiologically Controlled IVD	an IVD which may contain microorganisms which have been shown through process validation not to adversely affect product performance throughout the product's expected shelf life when stored according to the IVD's labeling.
Microbiologically Uncontrolled IVD	an IVD which contains components that are toxic to microorganisms or do not support the growth of microorganisms, and the remains or byproducts of any microorganisms in the IVD do not adversely affect product performance.
Retentive Filters	a filter placed in the process or product line to trap contaminants, where filter porosity may vary depending on the type of contaminants being retained.
Sterile	the complete absence of viable microorganisms from the product, as defined in USP, Section 1211.

Sterility Assurance
Level (SAL)

the probability of an item being non-
sterile, dependent on the product
bioburden and the lethality of the
sterilization process.

Sterile Filtered/
Sterilized by Filtration

IVDs which have been filtered through
a not greater than 0.22 micrometer or
smaller filter (which has been suitably challenged as per USP) either to
remove all viable microorganisms, or
to remove only certain types of microorganisms, and their production specifications and product labeling state:
1) the final filter pore size used; 2) the
specific viable microorganisms that
have been removed from the product
by filtration; and 3) the specific microorganisms whose absence has
been confirmed through testing of the
finished IVD.

Appendix D

A Compendium of Literature References on Validation for Medical Products

Agalloco, J. 1993. The Validation Life Cycle. *Journal of Parenteral Science and Technology,* May–June:142–147.

Agalloco, J. 1992. Points to Consider in the Validation of Equipment Cleaning Procedures. *Journal of Parenteral Science and Technology,* September/October:163–168.

ANSI/AAMI Guideline for Industrial EtO Sterilization of Medical Devices: Process Design, Validation, Routine Sterilization and Contract Sterilization. ST27-1988.

Carleton, F. J., and J. P. Agalloco. 1986. *Validation of Aseptic Pharmaceutical Processes.* New York: Marcel Dekker.

Chapman, K. G. 1991. A History of Validation in the United States: Part I. *Pharmaceutical Technology,* October:82–96.

Chapman, K. G. 1991. A History of Validation in the United States: Part II. *Pharmaceutical Technology,* November:54–70.

Commission of the European Communities. 1990. Analytical Validation. In *Rules Governing Medicinal Production in the European Community,* Volume IIIA. July:1–16.

DeSain, C. V. 1993. *Drug, Device and Diagnostic Manufacturing: The Ultimate Resource Handbook.* 2d ed. Buffalo Grove, IL: Interpharm Press.

DeSain, C. V. 1993. *Documentation Basics That Support Good Manufacturing Practices.* Cleveland: Advanstar Communications.

DeSain, C. V. 1992. Documentation Basics That Support Good Manufacturing Practices: Equipment and Utility System Validation Protocols. *BioPharm,* May:21–34.

DeSain, C. V. 1992. Documentation Basics That Support Good Manufacturing Practices: Master Method Validation Protocols. *BioPharm,* June:30–34.

DeSain, C. V. 1992. Documentation Basics That Support Good Manufacturing Practices: Process Validation Protocols. *BioPharm,* July–August:22–24.

DeSain, C. V., and C. L. Vercimak. 1994. *Implementing International GMPs for Drug, Device, and Diagnostic Manufacturers: A Practice Guide.* Buffalo Grove, IL: Interpharm Press.

DeVecchi, F. 1986. Validation of Air Systems Used in Parenteral Drug Manufacturing Facilities. In *Validation of Aseptic Pharmaceutical Processes,* F. J. Carleton and J. P. Agalloco, eds., pp. 125–162. New York: Marcel Dekker.

FDA. 1987. *Guidelines on the Principles of Process Validation.*

Finkelson, M. J. 1986. Validation of Analytical Methods by FDA Laboratories II. *Pharmaceutical Technology,* March:75, 78, 80–84.

Garfinkle, B. D. 1986. Validation of Utilities. In *Validation of Aseptic Pharmaceutical Processes,* F. J. Carleton and J. P. Agalloco, eds., pp. 185–205. New York: Marcel Dekker.

Guerra, J. 1986. Validation of Analytical Methods by FDA Laboratories I. *Pharmaceutical Technology,* March:74, 76, 78.

How Clean Is Clean?/Validation of Cleaning Procedures in Manufacturing Equipment. 1991. Bern: European Organisation for Quality.

Hudson, B. J., and L. Simmons. 1992. Streamlining Package-Seal Validation. *Medical Device and Diagnostic Industry,* October: 49–52, 89.

Morris, J. M. 1989. US and EEC Requirements for Documenting Process and Methods Validation. *Drug Information Journal,* Vol. 23:453–461.

Nally, J., and R. Kieffer. 1993. The Future of Validation: From QC/QA to TQ. *Pharmaceutical Technology,* October:106–116.

Stellon, R. C. 1986. Sterile Packaging Validation. *Medical Device and Diagnostic Industry,* October:42–46.

Sterilization of Health Care Products: Requirements for Validation and Routine Control: Gamma and Electron Beam Radiation Sterilization. ISO 11137-2.

Sterilization of Health Care Products: Requirements for Validation and Routine Control: Industrial Moist Heat Sterilization. ISO 11134.

Tetzlaff, R. F. 1993. Validation Issues for New Drug Development: Part III, Systematic Audit Techniques. *Pharmaceutical Technology,* January:80–88.

Tetzlaff, R. F., R. E. Shepherd, and A. J. LeBlanc. 1993. The Validation Story: Perspectives on the Systematic GMP Inspection Approach and Validation Development. *Pharmaceutical Technology,* March:100–116.

Validation of Compendial Methods. 1995. *U.S. Pharmacopeia 23,* Chapter 1225.

Validation of Dry Heat Processes Used for Sterilization and Depyrogenation. Technical Bulletin No. 3. Bethesda, MD: Parenteral Drug Association.

Validation and Routine Control of EtO Sterilization. ISO 11135.2.

Zeller, A. O. 1993. Cleaning Validation and Residue Limits: A Contribution to Current Discussions. *Pharmaceutical Technology,* October:70–80.

Appendix E

Additional Guideline Documents*

Association for the Advancement of Medical Instrumentation (AAMI)

AAMI Standard and Recommended Practices: Volume 2: Sterilization Equipment and Procedures, 4th Edition (1992)

Biological Indicators for Saturated Steam Sterilization in Health Care Facilities (1986)

Chemical Sterilants and Sterilization Methods—A Guide to Selection and Use (1990)

Determining Residual Ethylene Oxide in Medical Devices (1988)

Dosimetry for Monitoring Gamma Irradiation Sterilization of Medical Products (1989)

Guideline for Industrial Ethylene Oxide Sterilization of Medical Devices (1988)

Guideline for Industrial Moist Heat Sterilization of Medical Products (1987)

------

* For further information, availability, and price, write to Interpharm Press, Inc., 1358 Busch Parkway, Buffalo Grove, IL 60089-4515, U.S.A.

Process Control Guidelines for Gamma Radiation Sterilization of Medical Devices (1984)

International Organization for Standardization (ISO)

Code of Practice for Pharmaceutical Suppliers: Manufacture of Medicinal Products Contract Packaging Materials

Code of Practice for Pharmaceutical Suppliers: Manufacture of Pharmaceutical Raw Materials (Active Ingredients and Excipients)

Determination of Repeatability and Reproducibility for a Standard Test Method by Inter-Laboratory Tests (1986)

ISO 9000–International Standards for Quality Management, 3rd Edition (1993)

ISO 9000: Standards for Quality Systems—5 Volumes (1987)

ISO 9000-1—Guidelines for Selection and Use of Quality System Standards

ISO 9000-2—Guidelines for the Implementation of ISO 9001, 9002, 9003

ISO 9004-3—Quality Management and Quality System Elements: Guidelines for Processed Materials

ISO 9004-4—Quality Management and Quality System Elements: Guidelines for Quality Improvement

ISO 9004-6—Guidelines on Quality Planning

ISO 9004-7—Guidelines on Configuration Management

ISO 10011-1—Guidelines on Auditing Quality Systems Part 1: Auditing

ISO 10013—Guidelines for Developing Quality Manuals (CD 10013)

ISO 11134—Sterility of Healthcare Products: Requirements for Validation and Routine Control: Industrial Moist Heat Sterilization

ISO 11135.2—Medical Devices: Validation and Routine Control of Ethylene Oxide Sterilization

ISO 11137-2—Sterilization of Health Care Products: Validation and Routine Control: Gamma and Electron Beam Radiation Sterilization

9000—Quality Management and Quality Assurance Standards—Guidelines for Selection and Use (1987)

9000-3—Quality Management and Quality Assurance Standards—Part 3: Guidelines for the Application of ISO 9001 to the Development, Supply and Maintenance of Software (1991)

9001—Quality Systems—Model for Quality Assurance in Design/Development, Production, Installation and Servicing (1987)

9002—Quality Systems—Model for Quality Assurance in Production and Installation (1987)

9003—Quality Systems—Model for Quality Assurance in Final Inspection and Test (1987)

9004—Quality Management and Quality System Elements—Guidelines (1987)

Food and Drug Administration (US)

CDER

GMP General Guidelines/Drugs

Guidelines for the Validation of a Computerized Quality Control Data Management System

Biopharmaceutical Guidelines/Drugs

Guide for the Validation of Biological Indicators Incubation Time

Office of Generic Drugs Guides/Drugs

Method Validation for Compendial Drugs—Guide No. 90-12 (9/12)

FDA Inspection Technical Guides

Air Velocity Meters

Circular Temperature Recording Charts

The Computer in FDA Regulated Industries

Electronic Component Resistors, Temperature Sensors

EtO Sterilization

Evaluation of Production and Cleaning Processes for Devices—Contaminants, Cleaning Solvents

Expiration Dating and Stability Testing of Human Drugs

Heat Exchangers to Avoid Contamination

Hermetically Sealed Electronic Component Lead Detection

Industrial Application of Biochemical Technology

Leaking Test of Sealed Ampules for Parenteral Solutions

Lyophilization of Parenterals

Microbiological Contamination of Equipment Gaskets with Product Contact

Noise Control Mufflers for Bleeders or Sterilizers

Pyrogens and Bacterial Endotoxins

Radiation Protection Terminology

Reliability Testing of Manufactured Products

Screening Electronic Components by Burn-in

Steam Activated Heat Sensitive Sterilization Indicators

Steam Pressure Control for Retorts and Autoclaves

Texas Instruments TI-59 Programmable Calculator for Enforcement of X-ray Performance Standards

Thermocouples and Surface Pyrometers

Tin Whiskers in Medical Devices

Valves Used in Process Fluid Systems

Water for Pharmaceutical Use

CDRH/Medical Devices

Application of the Device Good Manufacturing Practice (GMP) Regulation to the Manufacture of Sterile Devices (2/83)

Application of the Medical Device GMP's to Computerized Devices and Manufacturing Processes—Medical Device Guidance for FDA (11/90)

Complete Blue Book—Office of Device Evaluation Guidance Memoranda (2/90)

Device Good Manufacturing Practices Manual; Fifth Edition—FDA 91-4179 (8/91)

Federal Standard: Clean Room and Work Station Requirements; Controlled Environments FED-STD-209D—Superseding . . . (6/88)

Good Laboratory Practice Regulations; Final Rule (9/87)

Guideline for the Manufacture of In-Vitro Diagnostic Products (1994)

Guideline of the Validation of the Limulus Amebocyte Lysate Test as an End-Product Endotoxin Test (12/87)

Guideline on General Principles of Process Validation (5/87)

Highlights of the 1990 Safe Medical Devices Act—FDA 91-4243

Inspections of Foreign Device Manufacturers (2/93)

Medical Device GMP Guidance for FDA Investigators (4/87)

A Pocket Guide to Device GMP Inspections—Inspections of Medical Device Manufacturers and GMP Regulation (11/91)

Points to Consider for Internal Reviews and Corrective Action Operating Plans; Availability and Fraud. Untrue Statements (9/91)

Pre-Production Quality Assurance Planning: Recommendations for Medical Device Manufacturers—FDA 90-4236 (9/89)

Product Development Protocol Guideline (11/80)

Shelf Life of Medical Devices (3/91)

Sterile Medical Devices: A GMP Workshop Manual; 4th Edition— FDA 84-4174 (1/85)

Appendix F

Information Sources

Agencies, Governmental

American National Standards
  Institute (ANSI)
11 West 42nd Street
New York, NY 10018 USA
212-642-4900
212-302-1286 Fax

CDRH, Office of Training and
  Assistance
**Division of Small Manufacturer's
  Assistance** (HFZ-220)
5600 Fishers Lane
Rockville, MD 20857
800-638-2041
301-443-6597
301-443-9435 Flash Fax

CDRH, Office of Device Evaluation
**Division of Reproductive,
  Abdominal, ENT and
  Radiological Devices**
1390 Piccard Drive, HFZ-402
Rockville, MD 20850
301-594-5072
301-594-2359 Fax

CDRH, Office of Device Evaluation
Division of Opthalmic Devices
1390 Piccard Drive, HFZ-460
Rockville, MD 20850
301-594-2205
301-594-2361 Fax

CDRH, Office of Device Evaluation
**Division of Clinical Laboratory
  Devices**
1390 Piccard Drive, HFZ-440
Rockville, MD 20850
301-594-3084
301-594-2360 Fax

CDRH, Office of Device Evaluation
**Division of Cardiovascular,
  Respiratory and Neurological
  Devices**
1390 Piccard Drive, HFZ-450
Rockville, MD 20850
301-594-2720
301-594-2361 Fax

CDRH, Office of Device Evaluation
**Division of General and
Restorative Devices**
1390 Piccard Drive, HFZ-410
Rockville, MD 20850
301-594-2036
301-594-2358 Fax

CDRH, Office of Compliance
Division of Bioresearch Monitoring
Oak Grove Corporate Center
2094 Gaither Road
Rockville, MD 20850
301-594-4718
301-594-4731 Fax

CDRH, Office of Compliance
Division of Enforcement I
Oak Grove Corporate Center
2094 Gaither Road
Rockville, MD 20850
301-594-4586
301-594-4636 Fax

CDRH, Office of Compliance
Division of Enforcement II
Oak Grove Corporate Center
2094 Gaither Road
Rockville, MD 20850
301-594-4611
301-594-4638 Fax

CDRH, Office of Compliance
Division of Enforcement III
Oak Grove Corporate Center
2094 Gaither Road
Rockville, MD 20850
301-594-4646
301-594-4672 Fax

CDRH, Office of Surveillance and
Biometrics
Division of Surveillance Systems
1390 Piccard Drive, HFZ-340
Rockville, MD 20850
301-594-1311
301-594-1996 Fax

CDRH, Office of Surveillance and
Biometrics
Division of Postmarket Evaluation
1390 Piccard Drive, HFZ-344
Rockville, MD 20850
301-594-2103
301-594-1996 Fax

CDRH, Office of Surveillance and
Biometrics
Division of Biometric Sciences
1390 Piccard Drive, HFZ-160
Rockville, MD 20850
301-594-0650
301-594-0050 Fax

CDRH
Office of Science and Technology
12720 Twinbrook Parkway, Bldg 5,
HFZ-100
Rockville, MD 20857
301-443-2444
301-443-2296 Fax

CDRH
**Office of Standards and
Regulations**
12720 Twinbrook Parkway, Bldg 5,
HFZ-80
Rockville, MD 20857
301-594-4762
301-594-4793 Fax

FDA **(HFR-2145) Region II**
850 Third Avenue
Brooklyn, NY 11232 USA
718-965-5043

FDA **(HFR-2245) Region II**
599 Delaware Avenue
Buffalo, NY 14202 USA
716-846-4483

FDA **(HFR-2345) Region II**
20 Evergreen Place
East Orange, NJ 07018 USA
201-645-3265

FDA **(HFR-2420) Region II**
Puerta de Tierra Station
P.O. Box 5719
San Juan 00906 **Puerto Rico**
819-753-4443

FDA **(HFR-3145) Region III**
US Customhouse, Room 900
2nd and Chestnut Streets
Philadelphia, PA 19106 USA
215-597-0837

FDA **(HFR-3245) Region III**
900 Madison Avenue
Baltimore, MD 21201 USA
301-962-3731

FDA **(HFR-3535) Region III**
1000 North Glebe Road, Room 743
Arlington, VA 22201 USA
703-285-2578

FDA **(HFR-4120) Region IV**
60 8th Street NE
Atlanta, GA 30309 USA
404-347-7355

FDA **(HFR-4220) Region IV**
7200 Lake Ellenor Drive #120
Orlando, FL 32809 USA
305-855-0900

FDA **(HFR-4320) Region IV**
297 Plus Park Boulevard
Nashville, TN 37217 USA
615-251-5028

FDA **(HFR-4575) Region IV**
6501 NW 36th Street #200
Miami, FL 33166 USA
305-526-2919

FDA **(HFR-5120) Region V**
433 West Van Buren Street
1222 Main Post Office
Chicago, IL 60607 USA
312-353-7126

FDA **(HFR-5245) Region V**
1141 Central Parkway
Cincinnati, OH 45202 USA
513-684-3501

FDA **(HFR-5345) Region V**
1560 East Jefferson Avenue
Detroit, MI 48207 USA
313-226-6260

FDA **(HFR-5445) Region V**
240 Hennepin Avenue
Minneapolis, MN 55401 USA
612-334-4100

FDA **(HFR-5525) Region V**
601 Rockwell Avenue #463
Cleveland, OH 44114 USA
216-522-4844

FDA **(HFR-5560) Region V**
575 North Pennsylvania
Indianapolis, IN 46204 USA
317-269-6500

FDA **(HFR-6145) Region VI**
1200 Main Tower Building 1545
Dallas, TX 75202 USA
214-767-5433

FDA **(HFR-6245) Region VI**
4298 Elysian Fields Avenue
New Orleans, LA 70122 USA
504-589-2420

FDA **(HFR-6345) Region VI**
Houston Station
1445 North Loop West #420
Houston, TX 77008 USA
713-229-3533

FDA **(HFR-6540) Region VI**
727 East Durango #B406
San Antonio, TX 78206 USA
512-229-6737

FDA (HFR-7245) Region VII
Laclede's Landing
808 North Collins Street
St. Louis, MO 63102 USA
314-425-5021

FDA (HFR-7515) Region VII
Brandeis Building
200 South 16th Street #430
Omaha, NE 68102 USA
402-221-4675

FDA (HFR-9145) Region IX
50 United Nations Plaza
San Francisco, CA 94102 USA
415-556-1457

FDA (HFR-9245) Region IX
1521 West Pico Boulevard
Los Angeles, CA 90015 USA
213-252-7597

FDA Administrative Office of Public Affairs
Electronic Bulletin Board
5600 Fishers Lane
Rockville, MD 20857 USA
800-222-0185
301-443-7318

FDA General Information
5600 Fishers Lane
Rockville, MD 20857 USA
301-443-1544

FDA/CBER
Congressional and Consumer Affairs
1401 Rockville Pike, HFM-12
Rockville, MD 20852
301-594-2000
301-594-1938 Fax

FDA/CDER
Legislative, Professional and Consumer Affairs
7520 Standish Place, HFB-008
Rockville, MD 20852
301-594-1012
301-594-3302 Fax

FDA/CDRH
1390 Piccard Drive
Rockville, MD 20850
800-638-2041
301-443-8818 Fax

National Institute of Standards and Technology
Gaithersburg, MD 20899 USA
301-975-4033

National Technical Information Service
US Department of Commerce
5285 Port Royal Road
Springfield, VA 22161 USA
703-487-4700
800-336-4700
703-321-8547 Fax

Journals, Newsletters, Periodic Reports*

Advances in Applied Biotechnology
Gulf Publishing Company

Applied Clinical Trials
Advanstar Communications

Beige Sheet: Technology Reimbursement Reports
FDC Reports, Inc.

Bio/Technology
Nature Publishing Company

BioPharm
AdvanstarPublications, Inc.

BioProcessing Technology
Technical Insights, Inc.

Biomedical Products
Gordon Publications, Inc.

Biotech Daily
Kings Publishing Group

Biotech Market News and Strategies
Vertis, Ltd.

Biotech Patent News

Biotechnology Law Report
Mary Ann Liebert, Inc.

Biotechnology Newswatch
McGraw-Hill, Inc.

Biotechnology Patent Digest
Mary Ann Liebert, Inc.

Biotechnology Progress, Journal of
 Food, Pharmaceutical and
 Bioengineering
Am. Inst. Chemical Engineers

Biotechnology in Japan Newsletter
Japan Pacific Associates

Blue Sheet: Health Policy and
 Biomedical Research
FDC Reports, Inc.

Chemical Week
American Chemical Society

Chemical and Engineering News
American Chemical Society

Clean Rooms
Witter Publishing Company

Commerce Business Daily: Federal
 Contract Awards Listing
Government Printing Office

Device and Diagnostic Regulator
Shotwell and Carr, Inc.

Devices and Diagnostic Letter
Washington Business Information

Dickinson's FDA Review Newsletter
Ferdic, Inc.

Drug Information Journal
Drug Information Association

Europe Drug and Device Report
Washington Business Information,
 Inc.

Europe Now: A Report
U.S. Department of Commerce

FDA Consumer
FDA

FDA Drug and Device Product
 Approvals
FDA, Freedom of Information
 Services

GMP Letter
Washington Business Information,
 Inc.

GMP Trends
P.O. Box 8001
Boulder, CO 80306 USA

Genetic Engineering News Magazine
Mary Ann Liebert, Inc.

Genetic Technology News
Technical Insights, Inc.

The Gold Sheet: Quality Control
 Reports
FDC Reports, Inc.

Gray Sheet: Medical Devices, Diag-
 nostics and Instrumentation
FDC Reports, Inc.

Green Sheet: Weekly Pharmacy
 Reports
FDC Reports, Inc.

Guide to Medical Device Regula-
 tion
Thompson Publishing Group

Hazardous Materials Transportation
Regulatory Bookshop

Hazardous Waste and Hazardous
 Materials
Mary Ann Liebert Publishers

In Vivo: The Business and Medicine
 Report
The Wilkerson Group

*International Pharmaceutical
Technology*
Advanstar Publications, Inc.

Journal of Biomaterials
Technomic Publishing Company

Journal of Irreproducible Results
Blackwell Scientific Publications

*Journal of Parenteral Science and
Technology*
Parenteral Drug Association

Journal of Pharmaceutical Science
American Pharmaceutical
Association

Laboratory Planning and Design
Advanstar Publishing Company

MDR Watch
Regulatory Bookshop

Machine Design Magazine
Penton Publishing

Medical Device Technology
Advanstar Publishing Company

*Medical Device and Diagnostic
Industry*
Canon Communications, Inc.

Medical Device Technology
Advanstar Communications

*Medical Products Manufacturing
News*
Canon Communications, Inc.

Microcontamination
Advanstar Publishing Company

Monoclonal Antibody News
Mary Ann Liebert, Inc.

NAmSA Update
North American Science Associates

Pharmaceutical & Biotech Daily
King Publishers

Pharmaceutical Digest
Centcom Publications

Pharmaceutical Engineering
International Society of
Pharmaceutical Engineers

Pharmaceutical Executive
Advanstar Publications, Inc.

Pharmaceutical Technology
Advanstar Publications, Inc.

*Pink Sheet: Prescription and OTC
Pharmaceuticals*
FDC Reports, Inc.

Plant Services
Putnam Publishing Company

*Power Magazine and The Power
Handbook*
McGraw Hill

Quality Engineering
Marcel Dekker, Inc.

Quality Progress
American Society for Quality
Control (ASQC)

Quality Systems Update
CEEM Information Service

RAPS Journal
RAPS

Regulatory Watchdog Service
Washington Business Information,
Inc.

*Rose Sheet: Toileteries, Fragrances
and Skin Care*
FDC Reports, Inc.

The Food and Drug Letter
Washington Business Information,
Inc.

Washington Drug Letter
Regulatory Bookshop

Publishers

Advanstar Communications
859 Willamette Street
Eugene, OR 97440
503-343-1200
503-343-3541 Fax

Advanstar Publications
7500 Old Oak Boulevard
Cleveland, OH 44130
800-598-6008
216-891-2726 Fax

American Institute of Chemical
　Engineers
345 East 47th Street
New York, NY 10017 USA
614-447-3776

American National Standards
Institute (ANSI)
11 West 42nd Street
New York, NY 10036
212-642-4900
212-302-1286 Fax

American Pharmaceutical
　Association
2215 Constitution Avenue NW
Washington, DC 20037 USA
202-628-4410

American Society of Quality Con-
　trol (ASQC)
611 East Wisconsin Avenue
Milwaukee, WI 53201
800-248-1946
414-272-8575
414-272-1734 Fax

Association for the Advancement
　of Medical Instrumentation
　(AAMI)
3330 Washington Boulevard
Suite 400
Arlington, VA 22201
800-332-2264
703-525-4890
703-276-0793 Fax

Blackwell Scientific Publications
3 Cambridge Center
Cambridge, MA 02142 USA
617-225-0401

Canon Communications, Inc.
3340 Ocean Park Boulevard
Santa Monica, CA 90405 USA
213-829-0315

CEEM Information Services
10521 Braddock Road
Fairfax, VA 22032-2231
703-250-5900
800-669-1567

Centcom, Ltd.
500 Post Road East
P.O. Box 231
Westport, CT 06881 USA

Drug Information Association
P.O. Box 3113
Maple Glen, PA 19002
215-628-2288
215-641-1229 Fax

FDC Reports, Inc.
5550 Friendship Boulevard
Chevy Chase, MD 20815 USA
301-657-9830
301-656-3094

Ferdic, Inc.
P.O. Box 367
Las Cruces, NM 88004-0367
505-527-8634
505-527-8858 Fax

GMP Trends
P.O. Box 8001
Boulder, CO 80306 USA

Gordon Publications, Inc.
301 Gibraltar Drive
Morris Plains, NJ 07950-0650 USA
201-292-5100
201-605-1220 Fax

Government Printing Office
732 North Capitol Street NW
Washington, DC 20402 USA
202-783-3238
202-512-2250 Fax

Gulf Publishing Company
P.O. Box 2608
Houston, TX 77252-2608 USA
713-529-4301
800-231-6275

International Society of Pharmaceutical Engineers (ISPE)
3816 West Linebaugh Avenue
Tampa, FL 33624 USA
813-960-2105
813-264-2816 Fax

Interpharm Press, Inc.
1358 Busch Parkway
Buffalo Grove, IL 60089
708-459-8480
708-459-6644 Fax

Japan Pacific Associates
467 Hamilton Avenue, Suite 2
Palo Alto, CA 94301 USA
415-322-8441

Kings Publishing Group
627 National Press Building
529 14th Street NW
Washington, DC 20077-1289 USA
202-638-4260
202-662-9719 Fax

Marcel Dekker, Inc.
270 Madison Avenue
New York, NY 10016 USA
212-696-9000
800-228-1160
914-796-1772 Fax

Mary Ann Liebert, Inc.
1651 Third Avenue
New York, NY 10130 USA
212-289-2300

McGraw Hill Publishers
1221 Avenue of the Americas
New York, NY 10020 USA
212-512-2000
800-262-4729

Nature Publishing Company
P.O. Box 1721
Riverton, NJ 08077 USA
800-524-0328

North American Science Associates (NAmSA)
2261 Tracy Road
Northwood, OH 43619 USA
419-666-9455

Parenteral Drug Association
7500 Old Georgetown Road #620
Bethesda, MD 20814
301-986-0293
301-986-0296 Fax

Penton Publishing
1111 Chester Avenue
Cleveland, OH 44114 USA
216-696-7000

Putnam Publishing Company
200 Madison Avenue
New York, NY 10016 USA
212-951-8400
800-631-8571

Regulatory Bookshop
1117 North 19th Street
Arlington, VA 22209-1798 USA
703-247-3434
800-426-3421
703-247-3421 Fax

Shotwell and Carr, Inc.
3003 LBJ Freeway
Dallas, TX 75234 USA
214-243-3567 Fax

Technical Insights, Inc.
P.O. Box 1304
Fort Lee, NJ 07024-9967 USA
201-568-4744
800-245-6217
201-568-8247 Fax

Technomic Publishing Company
851 New Holland Avenue
Box 3535
Lancaster, PA 17604 USA
717-291-5609
800-233-9936
717-295-4538 Fax

Thompson Publishing Group
1725 K Street NW
Washington, DC 20006
202-872-4000
800-925-1878

U.S. Department of Commerce
International Trade Administration
14th Street and Constitution Avenue
Washington, DC 20230 USA
202-377-5276

U.S. Pharmacopeial Convention
(USP)
12601 Twinbrook Parkway
Rockville, MD 20852
800-227-8772

Washington Business Information,
Inc.
1117 North 19th Street
Arlington, VA 22209 USA
800-426-0416
703-247-3421 Fax

Witter Publishing Company
84 Park Avenue
Flemington, NJ 08822 USA
201-788-0343

Index